Prospectives

~

Celebrating 40 Years of Associate Degree Nursing Education

D0967390

Prospectives

~

Celebrating 40 Years of Associate Degree Nursing Education

Jean Simmons
Editor

National League for Nursing Press • New York
Pub. No. 23-2517

ISBN 0-88737-576-6

The views expressed in this publication represent the views of the authors and do not necessarily reflect the official views of the National League for Nursing Press.

This book was typeset by Publications Development Company of Crockett, Texas. The editor and designer was Allan Graubard. Northeast Press was the printer and binder. The cover was designed by Lauren Stevens.

Printed in the United States of America

Contents

v

Contributors

Mary Ann Anderson, MS, RNC, CNA, Assistant Professor, Project Coordinator, Community College-Nursing Home Partnership, Weber State University, Ogden, UT.

Patricia M. Bentz, MSN, RN, Professor of Nursing, Shoreline Community College, Seattle, WA.

Mary Jo Boyer, MSN, RN, Assistant Dean and Director, Allied Health and Nursing, Delaware County Community College, Media, PA.

Ellen R. Bramoweth, MS, RN, CD, Instructor of Nursing, Mesa Community College, Mesa, AZ.

Gail Cobe, MSN, RN, Project Director, Community College-Nursing Home Partnership, Ohlone College, Fremont, CA.

Ivory C. Coleman, MS, RNC, Associate Professor, Department of Nursing, Community College of Philadelphia, Philadelphia, PA.

Janice R. Ellis, PhD, RN, Professor, Shoreline Community College, Seattle, WA.

Jean Flood, MSN, BSN, RN, Nursing Instructor, Northcentral Technical College, Associate Degree Nursing Program, Wausau, WI.

Carol Fountain, MN, RN, Associate Professor, Boise State University, Boise, ID.

Mary Beth Hanner, PhD, RNC, Dean, Nursing Programs, Regents College, Albany, NY.

Elizabeth J. Heywood, MS, RN, Nurse Educator/Program Associate, Regents College, Albany, NY.

Roberta Hunt, RN, BSN, MSPH, Instructor, Inver Hills Community College, Inver Grove, MN.

Marie J. Kaye, MS, RN, Nurse Educator/Program Associate, Regents College, Albany, NY.

Kathleen Lewis, MSN, RN, Nursing Instructor, Parkland College, Champaign, IL.

Claire Ligeikis-Clayton, MS, RN, BSN, CNS, Associate Professor/Chairperson, Nursing Department, Broome Community College, Binghamton, NY.

Carol Lillis, MSN, RN, Professor and Nursing Program Coordinator, Delaware County Community College, Media, PA.

Mary McKee, MED, RN, BSN, Dean of Community Services, Inver Hills-Lakewood Community Colleges, St. Paul, MN.

Vivian E. Ott, MSN, RN, Nursing Instructor, Roane State Community College, Harriman, TN.

Lynn Schneider, MSN, RN, BSN, Nursing Instructor, Northcentral Technical College, Associate Degree Nursing Program, Wausau, WI.

Jean Simmons, MSN, RN, Professor of Nursing, Greenfield Community College, Greenfield, MA.

Ellie Slette, MS, RN, BSN, Director of Nursing, Inver Hills-Lakewood Community Colleges, St. Paul, MN.

Emily T. Slunt, PhD, RN, Professor and Director, Nursing Education Program; Chairperson, Health Sciences Division, Howard Community College, Columbia, MD.

Pam Springer, MS, RN, Associate of Science Program Director, Boise State University, Boise, ID.

Eleanor L. Strang, PhD, RN, Director of Nursing, Central Arizona College, Coolidge, AZ.

Elaine Tagliareni, MS, RNC, Associate Professor, Community College of Philadelphia; Project Site Coordinator, Philadelphia; W.K. Kellogg, Community College Nursing Home Partnership Project, Philadelphia, PA.

Patricia Tymchyshyn, PhD, RN, Instructor and Curriculum Coordinator, Parkland College and University of Illinois, Champaign, IL.

Preface

Associate degree nursing education began in 1952 with three programs. Curricula have changed through the years, responding to health care needs of our population. Associate degree education, once thought of as "terminal" in nature, has become a pathway for educational and career mobility. The National League for Nursing Council of Associate Degree Programs is a professional association which acts as a national network of nurse educators who share interests, concerns and a passion for excellence in nursing education. To all who celebrate the past years of associate degree nursing education here is a publication that represents the enthusiasm of past experiences, the reflections of educators who truly enjoy the art and science of nursing, and curricular implementation designs currently in use.

The book is divided into four parts. Part I focuses on educational styles and concepts, including student-teacher relationships that reflect partnerships, standing "together," support measures for minority student success, and a nontraditional style of teaching content to the student of the 1990s.

Part II presents the unifying theme of empowering students. Chapters focus on critical thinking, total quality management and improvement, and implementation of a curriculum model reflective of a "caring" emphasis in today's educational domain.

Part III focuses on Associate Degree Nursing Education's response to the changing mode of health care delivery. Curriculum plans which meet the demands of health needs for those in community or long-term care settings and students' valuing caring for the elderly are discussed. Also included is a description of an exemplary preceptorship project as an appropriate model for long-term care.

Part IV concludes with examples of implementing computer usage "in" the classroom, including interactive video disc usage in the curriculum and a plan to integrate computer-assisted instruction that includes a 25-year review of the actual implementation of using computers in nursing education.

The conference from which this book arose, "Retrospectives, Intro-spectives and Prospectives: A Celebration of 40 Years of Associate De-gree Nursing Education," was held April 1992 in Phoenix, Arizona. This book is dedicated to Susan Sherman, CADP Meeting Chairperson, her enthusiasm and joy of nursing education inspired all of us.

Jean Simmons, MSN, RN, ADN (1965)

Foreword

*T*he year 1992 represented a milestone in the history of associate degree nursing—the 40th anniversary of its inception. April was a very special month for the NLN Council of Associate Degree Programs (CADP) as it was the national celebration of this anniversary. An ideal ambiance was provided by The Arizona Biltmore in Phoenix where nearly 450 educators, representing 43 states and the Commonwealth of Puerto Rico, gathered to reminisce about their rich heritage, celebrate their accomplishments, and chart their future.

While this annual meeting offered the many activities that our members have come to enjoy—impressive plenary sessions, lively business meetings, special social events, opportunities to network—this particular meeting can also boast of yet another milestone. For the first time in the Council's history, the Executive Committee called for abstracts with the hope that some of the members would take the opportunity to share their experiences and showcase their activities at this 40th anniversary celebration.

In response, more than 100 abstracts were submitted to the Program Committee for blind peer review and possible selection for presentation. Due to the outstanding quality of the abstracts, 18 breakout sessions were ultimately decided upon, considerably more than had originally been planned. In these 18 sessions there were a total of 31 presenters, 8 of whom are dean/directors of nursing programs, 3 program coordinators, and 20 faculty members.

All of the faculty members, and many of the administrators, identified themselves as teaching-team members or course leaders with a number of advisees, class and clinical responsibilities, and a portion of their out-of-classroom time committed to curriculum work and involvement in college-wide committees.

The majority of these presenters held membership in their professional organizations—ANA, NLN, and Sigma Theta Tau—were NLN site visitors and some had even served on the CADP Board of

Review. All had either published, conducted research, presented at national and regional meetings, or had written grants. A few held specialty certification and several had received their first nursing degree in the associate degree program where they presently hold faculty positions.

Each of the breakout sessions presented by these associate degree educators was hallmarked by creative, cutting edge and practical solutions to the challenges that face nurse educators in the 1990s—improving student faculty relationships, addressing community-based learning, incorporating high-technology, and enhancing critical thinking skills, to mention only a few.

A special tribute is due to the members of the Council's Executive Committee and Program Committee who had the faith in the Council membership to challenge them to share their accomplishments and a special tribute to the members who responded to that challenge.

Gratitude goes to all of those who not only presented in Phoenix but have shared their presentations here in written form. To all of you who have not yet presented your work at a national meeting, perhaps you will be inspired to respond to a future Council Call for Abstracts.

Barbara Murphy, EdD, RN
Vice President for Council Affairs
Director, Council of Associate Degree Programs
National League for Nursing

PART I

Educational Styles and Concepts

1

Prospectives: Creating the Future
The Story of a Teacher-Student Partnership

Elaine Tagliareni

*L*ast Thursday, just before coming here to Phoenix, I said good-bye to my clinical group of graduating fourth-semester students. It was their last clinical day. Although I've done that every spring for the past 13 years now, I always have mixed feelings. I thought about the tentative individuals I had nurtured through fundamentals. As I saw them take their leave, however, I was dazzled by the confidence that stemmed from their greater sense of themselves that grew from a keen understanding of their work as individuals and well-developed nursing skills.

That's what teaching in Associate Degree nursing is all about. Being with students, knowing them, learning with them, watching them grow over time, all make our job as educators so special. That, too, is the subject of this chapter. Really what I want to talk with you is the power of the teacher-student relationship, the transforming nature of that relationship, and the creation of a future by being fully present with students as we educate them.

I've never been really big on predicting the future. You see, I took a class as an undergraduate, taught by a philosopher who billed himself as a futurist. I thought to myself, "I'll take this course, find out what will happen over the next 20 years, and plan my life around it." The first two sessions started rather slowly, and the next 43 sessions never really picked up. We talked about the past and the present, not much about the future. I remember one gray winter afternoon, as I was beginning to nod off during class, a friend poked me and said, "Elaine, I'd wake up if I were you; he's about to predict World War II!" Actually, I learned a great deal in that class. I learned that predicting the future, as an exercise, has its limitations; you are there by the time you have figured it out. The truth is, we consult our past for guidance, but the choices we make today, right now, are always an adventure that takes us into the future. What I do today will shape and create the future— in that way, the now takes on a special significance. At least I learned that from the futurist. Since then, over the years, I've come to appreciate the present even more. We bring meaning to our lives and to the world by being fully present with others today. I know the world only through my involvement with it now.

Now, mind you, the past also plays a significant part. We cannot worship the past nor can we ignore it; rather, we must capture the spirit of the past in order to see the future more clearly. And ours is a past, 40 years old, filled with innovation and expansion, a past ripe with adventure and creativity. We sit here today, in beautiful Phoenix, enjoying the fruits of experimentation and the imaginative decision making of the 1950s and the 1960s. I am proud to be an Associate Degree Educator and part of this rich and innovative heritage. The development of programs to educate nurses in the Community College changed all of nursing forever. The curriculum, the students, and the learning activities were dramatically unlike other nursing programs at the time.

Verle Waters tells a story about those early days:

> *As a new teacher in that strange new program, I came on the ward with twelve students ranging in age from 17 to 58, including two men. I said, "We'll be here until noon, we'll have post-conference and then we'll leave. We'll do these baths and treatments, but we won't do those, because they don't fit our learning objectives this week." The head nurse looked at me and my students of assorted sex, age and shape like we were aliens from another planet. The prevailing opinion was that the students would be no good. How could they be without eight weeks of night duty? How can you still learn if you're a grandmother? If they did graduate, because of our loose standards,*

they certainly would not pass the licensing examination. Many thought the experiment would end as quickly as it had arisen. But the programs endured and thrived. (Waters, 1992)

The introduction of pre- and post-conference, use of weekly practice records instead of mammoth case studies, the integrated curriculum, all of these "experiments" originated in Associate Degree Nursing Education; all of these "experiments" have become the norm in nursing education today.

The students themselves looked different in those early programs. No nursing teacher before had encountered the challenge of such diversity: students ranging in age from 16 to 59 years, veterans, culturally diverse, men and women, married or divorced with children; they lived at home and commuted to school. An entirely new population of talented, ambitious, committed people came into nursing.

Last Thursday, I walked with that group of talented, ambitious, committed people to the parking garage on their last day of clinical experience. I looked at them and said to myself, "They are our future but they are also our link with the past." Students help us capture the spirit of our past, a past exemplified by innovation, creativity, and an unbounding desire to be different, a past characterized by growth and diversity. And I knew, last Thursday, as I have always known, that if we live more fully in the present with our students, together as partners, that is our future. The future, like the past 40 years, belongs solely to us. It is ours to fashion, to mold, not to react to, but to create. And we create that future by being present with students today, helping them to discover who they are and what they can become within the context of the nursing experience. By being open and fully present in a meaningful way with students today, the future will unfold, and like our past, it will be dynamic and visionary.

I have several ideas about how to make that happen. In 1989, at the National League for Nursing sponsored Nurse Educator Conference in Philadelphia, Janet Quinn spoke about the four principles of an effective teacher-student relationship. Since then, I've reflected on those principles, expanded on them, and put my own twist on them.

SHOW UP

The first principle is simply, show up! But, showing up is not all that easy, you know.

My favorite showing up story is actually my husband's story. My husband, Sal, does a great deal of public speaking. Several years ago, a Senior Citizens Group at our local church asked him to be a speaker at their Annual Communion Breakfast. Sal worked very hard at preparing his speech. He wanted to tell them about the valuable contribution they have made to society, boost their self-esteem, give them some ideas about how their lives have meaning now. When he stood up to speak, everybody clapped politely. And as he spoke he felt pretty good about what he was saying and about how his words would be interpreted by his listeners. After he had spoken for about ten minutes, in a stage whisper right in front of him at one of the tables, he heard these words, "Is the speaker here yet?" Needless to say, Sal wrapped up very quickly. As he left the stage, the women thanked him profusely, and told him how meaningful his words were. Rest assured, that as a public speaker Sal never again took himself quite so seriously.

I'm particularly fond of this story; actually, it has helped me put the "show up" business into perspective. Like you, I try to show up, to be there for students, to care about them and spend time with them. But showing up is complicated. You see, showing up means we are willing to be changed by the experience, willing to grow and find meaning in every teacher-student encounter, willing not to settle for what seems the inevitable. Showing up involves the determination to keep trying, no matter how skeptical you may feel.

I'm reminded again of a clinical day I spent at Greenfield Community College. I had a student who rarely showed initiative; in fact, this particular student followed me around like a wounded puppy dog. So I decided to show up for her and talk to her one day about how she could be more assertive in the clinical setting. I met her in the Conference Room and we talked at length about how she could act differently. It was one of those days when I felt that I was particularly brilliant. We've all had those days, haven't we? The student and I role played together; we talked about how this kind of behavior was probably part of her past experience and she left that Conference Room saying, "I understand, Elaine, I need to take charge, I'm going to be different now." I left that Conference Room thinking to myself, "You're really pretty good, Elaine. They don't pay you enough." Together we returned to the unit and the student said to me, "I think I'll go check my patient." Within two minutes she was back at my side. "Elaine," she said, "I need to speak with you." I thought to myself, "My, more insight, I don't know if I can handle this." She said to me, "Elaine, my patient is asleep, what should I do now?" I thought to myself, "Is the speaker here yet?"

Showing up takes time and patience. Giving up is the antithesis. Additionally, showing up requires energy, tremendous energy. But the essence of showing up involves realizing what value we bring to the process and there is no substitute for what we can bring to the teacher-student relationship—none. When we treat ourselves as valued persons, when we recognize the energy, the experience, the value we bring to each student encounter, when we treat our students as valued participants, that's value-added teaching. Value-added teaching means that in the process of teaching nursing we help the students to value themselves. Value-added teaching is the key to showing up.

Last fall, I met my seminar group in fundamentals, just as many of you did. We introduced ourselves and I listened to their stories. Karen has four children under the age of nine; her husband left and offers her no support. "It means the world to me," she said, "to be here in this program." Gail is 49 years old. Her daughter finished college last year—now it's Gail's turn. Grace, recently immigrated from Jamaica, said, "I'm going back. My country is so poor and nurses make such a difference there." Joe, who has worked as a security guard for 15 years, has three kids. The kids are all supportive of his nursing school adventure and Joe continues to work full-time. The commitment and diversity in that room captured me. I thought to myself, "I need to show up for these individuals."

In late November, Karen, the student with the four children, came to me and said, "I need to quit. My day care is unreliable and my part-time job just doesn't cover our expenses." I brought her to see the program director, and together we sought resources for Karen. She was able to stay in the program. Karen stopped by my office one week later. "You know, Elaine," she said, "I thought you would agree that I should quit. Thanks for not giving up on me."

We hear that all the time from our students. What they are really saying is, "Thank you for not giving up on me when I had given up on myself." Value-added teaching compels us to change that message. Henry Ford was fond of saying, "Whether you think you can or can't, you're right." Showing up is adding value to the teacher-student encounter; showing up is helping students believe they can!

BE ATTENTIVE

The second principle is be attentive. Being attentive really has to do with listening well.

My favorite listening well experience belongs to my Aunt Josie. One day, a few years ago, I drove Aunt Josie and Cousin Annie, her contemporary, to my home, about a 90-minute trip. They sat in the back seat. As we worked our way down the turnpike, Cousin Annie talked continuously about one tragedy after another. "Cousin Pete had another nervous breakdown; Cousin Martha's daughter has a terminal disease and her husband left her two days before her daughter's wedding; my children didn't call me on my birthday; they don't love me anymore; my arthritis is acting up." It's a shame that a plot writer from "All My Children" wasn't in the car; he could have taken the rest of the year off! Throughout the entire ride, Aunt Josie said nothing; however, she nodded her head appropriately at specific times. After one solid hour, Cousin Annie finally drew a breath. Aunt Josie leaned toward her, grasped Cousin Annie's hand, and said, in Italian, "What are you gonna do?"

I learned a great deal about listening that day. Cousin Annie didn't want solutions or helpful suggestions. Culturally it was acceptable behavior to carry on and then be done with it. Aunt Josie knew that; she listened well and this is the key to being attentive. Aunt Josie understood Cousin Annie's world. For those of us in Associate Degree Nursing Education, listening well takes on a special significance. The diversity of our student population compels us to listen within the context of the student, within the context of the environment and the culture from which the student comes, not to listen according to our own agenda or our own experience. Being sensitive to a world that I may never have witnessed or known is what being attentive is all about.

When Robert, another student in my seminar group, came to tell me that he had missed another class, I asked why. Robert had already been absent two times. He told me that he was unable to be in class because he had an appointment with his caseworker that day and that he had to be at the appointment to reestablish his medical benefits. I was about to answer from the context of my world which says, "If there is a conflict, call and change the appointment to another day." But Robert's world is very different from mine. Robert's world gives a quite different message to its inhabitants. Robert said to me, "If you don't come to welfare when you are assigned, you may go to the bottom of the list and then my family would have no health care." At that moment I listened differently to Robert. Understanding within the context of Robert's experiences told me that in this situation he made the right decision to miss class. I hope I will always remember that encounter with Robert.

Being sensitive to diversity doesn't mean giving up our standards regarding attendance or responsible conduct, and it also does not mean asking the student to conform to our world in every encounter, with every decision. Being attentive means valuing both worlds. Being attentive means helping students understand that they are listened to for who they are and what they are now, not who they will become someday.

Many of us during this conference have provided models to meet the challenge of cultural diversity. We need to expand and amplify that work. Being attentive, championing the diversity that is so much a part of our history, means listening according to the context of the student's background and cultural norms. That sensitivity and awareness must be a part of our future.

TELL THE TRUTH

The third principle, tell the truth, might also be termed tough love. Telling the truth doesn't just mean giving less than positive feedback or praise, but telling the truth always means being honest. And yet telling the truth means more than that.

When we tell the truth, we bring to the students the inherent belief that they have value. It's important here to make the distinction between self-worth and worthiness. Self-worth fluctuates based on circumstances: a bad day in skills lab, difficulty with a personal relationship, a C on a test when an A was expected. But the worthiness of an individual doesn't change day-to-day; all human persons have inherent worthiness. For our students, we are a bridge to recognition of their worthiness. So often when we tell the truth, we need to point out deficits; it's the nature of our work. We give students prescriptions to employ to be successful, and sometimes those prescriptions are difficult and unpopular. By telling the truth, we raise the bar on their performance, challenging them, encouraging them, critiquing them, refreshing them. Telling the truth is a process enhanced by collegial, egalitarian relationships between student and teacher. Yesterday, for instance, Em Bevis spoke about establishing a climate of sorority and fraternity, of equality and dialogue between student and teacher in a caring, educative curriculum; telling the truth thrives in this climate. Sadly, so often in our history, the traditional, behaviorally based model of teacher-student interactions has deflated and stymied the process of ensuring worthiness.

When I first met Sal's mother, Grandma Tag, I was at a traditional family Sunday dinner. Everyone in the family was there—30 intimate relatives. The conversation turned to Uncle Frank, the family black sheep—every family has at least one! The entire family held a lively discussion about how Frank confiscated canned goods from railroad cars and sold them in his grocery store, how he didn't come visit Grandpa on his deathbed, how he gambled away the grocery money. I noticed Grandma said nothing throughout the entire "anti-Frank" discussion. Finally, after she finished serving the meal, she sat next to me and said, "Elaine, I want you to know something about Frank. Frank is an excellent whistler."

I told that story to a new faculty member just the other day. She had come to my office for help in writing a clinical warning, her first. She had agonized over the decision to fail the student. The student was Gail, you remember, the seminar student who was taking "her turn." The faculty member liked Gail; she appreciated her commitment to nursing and the energy she expended to be a professional, at long last. But she knew, based on numerous clinical incidents, that Gail was not ready to move on. When I told her the whistling story, she listened politely and finally said, "Cute story, Elaine, but what does that story have to do with Gail and writing a clinical failure?" "Actually," I said, "it has everything to do with it." In this moment, telling the truth meant that Gail would not continue in the program. But telling the truth means ensuring worthiness. "When Gail leaves," I said to that faculty member, "knowing that for now she has not succeeded in nursing, we owe her the knowledge that she is valued and that she has inherent worthiness. At the very least," I said, "we must send her off believing that she is one excellent whistler."

ACCEPT WHAT HAPPENS

The final principle, accept what happens, may be my favorite. To accept what happens means not being attached to the outcome. It is not, however, a decision to be mediocre.

Not being attached to the outcome has a great deal to do with valuing students' ability and willingness to embrace the educational process. It has a great deal to do with grounding our curricula in "being in the world." Curriculum lives when it takes place in the context of reality, or as Bevis and Murray (1990, p. 328) tell us, "Schooling is not preparation for life; it is life."

The licensed practical nurse (LPN) accelerated class at the Community College of Philadelphia taught me so much about this living curriculum. LPN students are a wonderful group with lots to say in class. They come to school with a wealth of clinical experience. One day last fall I practiced, "The students aren't going to do well on the next test. They had so much to contribute in class, so many examples, that I didn't say everything in my notes." The students, as you can guess, did just fine on the test.

I learned a great deal from that moment. Accepting what happens, giving directions to the flow of information, presenting myself, the teacher, as the expert colleague, rather than as the sole surveyor of knowledge, changes the way I view teaching and requires a rethinking of what learning is. Bevis and Murray (1990) describe learning in the educative-caring curriculum model as not merely acquiring knowledge or gathering and correlating facts, but as seeing the significance of life as a whole, discovering lasting values, relating learning to personal, reality-based experience. Who but you and I, who teach nursing every day to adult learners with a wealth of personal experiences, students who understand, sometimes far better than I, the realities of life and living, who but you and I are better positioned to teach in this emancipatory style? And yet, accepting what happens, promoting student learning that involves active engagement of students and includes collaboration with teachers and commitment to reality and lived experience, has not traditionally been a part of our comfort zone.

Freire (1970) described the predominant mode of teaching as the "banking process" of education, where students are viewed as the depositories and the teacher issues communiqués and makes deposits that the students receive, memorize, and repeat. Freire maintains that we must rethink a paradigm where the teacher teaches, thinks, talks, disciplines, chooses, acts, selects the content, has the authority, and is the subject of the learning process. We must rethink the paradigm where students are taught, know nothing, accept the teacher's thoughts, listen, are corrected, comply, have the illusion of acting, and hold the magical belief that we, the teachers, are the sole disciples of truth.

Accepting what happens, as an essential principle of the teacher-student relationship, demands that we value the ability of the student to learn, that we change the fundamental relationship between and among teachers and students. It's not easy. I still obsess about what content I've missed. Every day when I drive home from clinical, I think about what else I should have done, what I should have emphasized, how I will correct it tomorrow. The decision for excellence drives us in our daily work with students. But after all is said and done, we can't control what happens. We can't predict the events that will shape the students' experiences. But if we design our curricula well, with clear objectives that give focus to our teaching-learning activities, then we can be less prescriptive about the outcome. Accepting what happens means not being so attached to the outcome that we can't see or hear the learning that truly emerges. Bonner (1965) said that experience must be taken as it comes, at its face value and in its living form. When we ground curriculum in reality, in reflection, in everyday events, we help students to frame their learning, their care-planning decisions, and their understanding of themselves as nurses within the context of their lives. This mandate belongs to you and me. For 40 years, students with a variety of backgrounds and life experiences, mature students with a sincere commitment to learning and to nursing, have knocked on our door. They have showed up and listened attentively to us. We now owe them a relationship with us, their teachers, that is egalitarian and collaborative. Our future depends on it.

But accepting what happens is not limited to our relationship with students. Accepting what happens also involves rethinking what we teach, accepting the present, and understanding the world in which we practice nursing today as it is, not as we envision it in some ill-defined future. Strangely enough, this sounds like a job for my old teacher, the futurist! If he were here, and thank your lucky stars that he isn't, the scenario might unfold like this: He would predict that we have entered the age of degenerative disease, where individuals with four or more chronic illnesses are the major recipients of nursing care. He would say that the population is aging, that more and more older Americans require restorative as well as maintenance care, and that these individuals constitute 75 percent of a nurse's work. He could add that the AIDS epidemic is here to stay and has become the 15th leading cause of death in the United States and that infant mortality is staggeringly high due to inadequate prenatal care resulting from drugs and poverty. Then you would say cynically, "That's not in the future, that's happening right now in my community." And I would add, "If that's so, do our curricula, today, right now, prepare students to be competent, knowledge-based health care practitioners with older adults, with individuals with AIDS, and with young mothers who may be addicted and poor? Do our curricula teach students to value maintenance of optimal functional ability and to seek rehabilitation potentials despite chronic illnesses? Do they teach the practice of patterns that are critical to effective, responsive care for older adults?"

Next, our futurist would predict that issues related to quality of life, extension of life, and dying are becoming more complicated. He would predict that the basic rule so often followed in the health care arena, to extend life using all measures, doesn't work in all settings as patients, families, and society explore more complex issues involving the definition of death, the patient's wishes for autonomy and self-determination and the equitable distribution of society's resources. And you would call out in frustration, "That's not in the future, that's happening right now." So I ask you, "If that's so, do our curricula, right now, address these issues? Do the clinical experiences we choose for our students assist them to encounter these issues in their day-to-day practice? How do we provide opportunities for meaningful dialogue about ethical imperatives implicit in day-to-day practice?"

Last, our futurist would predict that the hospital has become a transition place, not a landing place for cure. He would say that the past three decades have witnessed an amazing growth in diagnostic and therapeutic capabilities brought about by technology, and that a health care system driven by technology will further depersonalize care and fragment it into a series of short-term encounters with a growing number of technologically oriented, specialized providers. "Oh that's happened already," you call out. And I would ask, "Do our curricula, right now, account for these changes? Do we help students to understand the high-technology, high-stimulus, fast-paced environment of acute care? Do we place too heavy an emphasis on individualization of care planning while they are there? Are our expectations realistic? Do we provide students with opportunities to know clients over time, to evaluate nursing care decisions, to be healers, to make connections, to understand and value the mission of nursing in a world seized by technology?" As the scenario unfolds, the message becomes a mandate. The futurist's predictions are not in the future, but the present. We have only to open our eyes and listen more intently. We have only to accept what has already happened. The future is right here, with us, all around us. As we open ourselves to it, we will see it more clearly and accept its vision. There is an old saying on Wall Street, "To know and not to do, is not to know." Creating the future involves knowing the present and living fully in the present with our students as they encounter the world of health care.

The future is right here among us today. We are our future. The students are our future. The future sits in front of us every day in the classroom. The future works with us, side-by-side, in the clinical setting. I left the future last Thursday in that parking garage in Philadelphia. Our alliance with our students in educational relationships is a partnership that has shaped our past, a past rich in innovation, creativity, and responsiveness, and it is that same partnership that will take us down the untraveled road, once again.

To quote Verle Waters again, "We are the experiment that came to stay." For 40 years we have showed up and made a difference in the lives of our students, teaching them nursing but at the same time, through the transforming nature of the student-teacher relationship, creating fulfillment and possibility. Verle Waters (1992) spoke recently about this legacy. She stated, "This July more than 40,000 men and women, young and not-so-young, short and tall, white and non-white, just your average bunch of smart, motivated, ambitious folks will graduate from Associate Degree programs and sit for the N-CLEX RN exam and take jobs across the country providing caring, competent nursing care to individuals who require their care and support." This is a powerful legacy.

When people ask me what I am most proud of in my life, I tell them that I am proud of my family. That's probably why I wanted you to meet them today, to know Sal, Grandma, and Aunt Josie, because my family has a lot do to with who I am and what I have become. But I also tell those who will listen, what else I am most proud of in my life. I tell them that I am proud to be an Associate Degree Nursing Educator, to be part of the legacy of Associate Degree Nursing because, quite honestly, my professional family has a lot to do with who I am and what I have become. As teachers, we are touched daily by diversity, commitment, and visions of what is to be. Our work impacts profoundly on the lives of women and men who come to us within the context of the nursing experience and we make a difference in their lives, insuring worthiness, valuing them. Like you, I am proud of this role. The story of the teacher-student relationship in Associate Degree Nursing Education is one of transformation and possibility.

We are a family, you and I, with our students. And like any family group who wants only good things for its members, we have a dream to build and hopes to fulfill. Like any family built solidly on its historical traditions and past successes, we will survive and thrive, stronger and wiser, by living fully in the present with our faces turned toward the future. We are a family growing stronger, growing wiser, growing free. For 40 years we have showed up. For the next 40 years and beyond, we will continue to be the speaker who shows up, listens, accepts what has happened, insures worthiness and value, and celebrates our educational relationships with students.

Feel good about what you do, about what you accomplish every day. We are incredible teachers, you and I. When this text is ended, clap not for me, but do not appreciate its author as much as the educator, your colleague, you work beside. For your colleague is a very special teacher who is part of a movement that transformed nursing education. We have so much to be proud of, you and I. In the powerful play "A Man for All Seasons," Sir Thomas More says to Master Rich, "You'd be a fine teacher, perhaps even a great one." "And if I was," replies Master Rich, "who would know it?" Sir Thomas More answers, "You would know it; your pupils would know it, your friends would know it and God" (Bott, 1960). And that, readers, is one incredible audience!

REFERENCES

Bevis, E.O., & Murray, J. (1990). The essence of the curriculum revolution: Emancipatory teaching. *Journal of Nursing Education, 29*(7).

Bonner, H. (1965). *On being mindful of man.* Boston: Houghton Mifflin.

Bott, R. (1960). *A man for all seasons.* New York: Vintage Books.

Freire, P. (1970). *Pedagogy of the oppressed.* New York: Herder and Herder.

Waters, V. (1992, March). Speech presented at Northampton Community College, Bethlehem, Pennsylvania.

2

The Success Project: A Model to Increase Admission, Retention, and Graduation of Minority Students

Ivory C. Coleman

A lthough barriers to minority student access and success in nursing curricula have been identified frequently in the nursing literature, exploration and evaluation of effective interventions have not received the same intensity of study. The need to focus on specific interventions that work in an urban community college is critical if nursing education hopes to increase minority student success.

The Success Project at Community College of Philadelphia attempted to address the nursing shortage and future supply of nurses by targeting minorities, specifically African American and Hispanic females, for social support and analytic skill building. The project identified 12 students who had successfully completed one semester (9–12 credits) of pre-college developmental coursework in reading, writing, and mathematics. Using individual education plans developed for each student, the project provided customized interventions and support services. In this chapter, I discuss insights and lessons learned for faculty with similar goals.

THE SELECTION PROCESS

A self-identification process in conjunction with college placement testing, where students are designated ESL or pre-college, was used to identify 30 potential nursing students who were then contacted by mail and invited to participate. Students were followed by the Office of Health Careers Opportunity (OHCO) and the project director to coordinate appropriate academic support, counseling, academic advising, and career exploration. Twelve students expressed interest in the Success Project.

SOCIAL SUPPORT ACTIVITIES

An assessment was made of each student's need for social and academic support, and individual counseling was offered. It is significant to note that even when provided with opportunity for appropriate social and academic support, the majority of students were not successful. For example, Jackie, an African American female approximately 27 years of age, had two children and was recently divorced. Jackie had successfully completed several non-science courses. She felt ready to begin the science pre-nursing sequence and the project director, along with OHCO director, agreed that she should take Biology 101. From the beginning, Jackie engaged in the right learning activities: she met with the teacher to discuss any questions or concerns she had about the course material; she sought tutoring from the Learning Laboratory; and she went to the biology tutorial laboratory. She failed the first two examinations. After each examination, she understood the course material. The support team discussed her difficulties with the instructor and followed that discussion with an individual conference, noting in a positive way that Jackie had participated in all tutorial activities. Prior to the third test the support team talked with Jackie about the upcoming examination. She stated, "I feel well prepared." Although Jackie did better in this examination than in the prior two, she still did not pass. Subsequently, she withdrew from the course and severed her ties with the project. None of the support services designed to assist Jackie was effective. Is there a problem, then, with the system or with the career choice?

Throughout the academic year, three support workshops were offered. One workshop involved offering support in an area of known barriers to academic success such as time management, management of credit load, management of personal and family responsibilities, goal setting, and financial planning. For this workshop, letters of invitation were mailed to the 12 students, and an RSVP was requested. Refreshments were available. It was a rainy evening and only one student attended. At a second meeting designed to introduce the students to their minority support person or "cheerleader," attendance again was poor. Only one African American student came to meet the six volunteer cheerleaders, one from the local Black Nurses Association and five from local chapter of Chi Eta Phi sorority.

The recruitment of minority nurse advocates had been the easiest task. Generally, minority organizations have as a central purpose the fostering of educational aspirations and achievement, and readily commit to programs that offer such support opportunities. Unfortunately, the minority cheerleaders, while attempting to contact their identified student, met with discouraging results. One cheerleader was told that the student was too busy to talk and to call later. The cheerleader was quite upset about the student's response, and needed assurance from the project director that this was a normal response and that the student would probably contact her. Attempts were also made to match the students with the cheerleader based on some common interest. In this case, they were from the same areas of the city. Another issue was the frequency of telephone number changes by students, producing a problem for cheerleaders as they attempted to contact their assigned student.

ANALYTIC SKILL-BUILDING ACTIVITIES

Community College of Philadelphia has an excellent support program through the Division of Educational Support Sciences, providing specialized assistance to students in reading, writing, and mathematics. Nursing students must be eligible for college level courses in these areas as a condition of acceptance into the curriculum.

One week noncredit pre-science workshops were offered to introduce beginning knowledge and study skills for introductory biology and chemistry courses. These workshops, offered by the Division of Educational Resource Services, are designed to decrease anxiety about science courses. All of the students involved in the project encountered difficulty in enrolling in these pre-semester workshops because the courses were over-subscribed or occurred at perceived unacceptable times.

BARRIERS TO SUCCESS

A major difficulty for students is the amount of time it will take for them to complete the pre-nursing coursework and be ready to enroll in the nursing curriculum. Time factors must clearly be understood from the beginning. Each individual student's educational plan, semester by semester, should be clearly mapped. Initially, while this group of students accepted the extended time frame, it later became a source of discouragement. At this point, one of the primary tasks of the cheerleader emerges: the "rah rah" speech and continued encouragement to persist.

Financial aid may represent another barrier for students. Many students have defaulted on previous college loans and are ineligible for additional aid. The financial aid office worked out payment plans as students waited for aid to be approved, but students did not always fully understand the commitment this entails. For example, Delores had defaulted on two loans from two different institutions. Although Delores pays money regularly on her defaulted loans, the regulator did not feel that substantial payment had been made and would not approve a new loan. The financial aid officer at the college was attempting to assist Delores by allowing her to pay in installments for a course. Delores started classes and attended for seven weeks. She began searching for a less expensive 3-credit course over her present 4-credit course. She withdrew from the approved 4-credit course and registered for the 3-credit course. Delores made this decision without discussing it with the project director or the financial aid officer. The financial aid officer discovered her course change and withdrew her. Delores and the project director spent hours discussing this process, because she could not understand that changing courses without prior approval was a problem. The project director pointed out the original agreement and how the rules had been set to assist her. This problem was never resolved to Delores' satisfaction. However, she is taking another course and is determined to be a nurse.

Family responsibilities represents another barrier. Many students involved in the project have small children and need to manage their dependents' education along with their own. This presents problems to the potential student as it relates to course schedules, meeting with the project chair, or their cheerleader.

RESULTS AND CONCLUSIONS

The project staff have identified the following items as points of concern in the successful pursuit of minority students, in this case African American and Hispanic females, for nursing careers:

- Students can be supported to seek and use appropriate advising and academic support.
- Minority nurse advocates were identified and linked to the minority student. Minority nurse advocates were trained to be cheerleaders, and were available to provide "rah rah" speeches. They were not responsible for the student's academic areas.
- Many students have academic difficulty with the pre-college coursework even though all available support programs have been engaged.
- A support team that involved the Department Head of Nursing, the project director, an allied health counselor, a reading specialist, and the director of the Office of Health Careers Opportunity, was formed. This group has assisted in the evaluation of the project and made the following recommendations:

    —Choose a target population of students with stronger academic skills because the group chosen may not have the academic skills to accomplish their goals.

    —Talk to faculty in the developmental programs and have them make recommendations about potential students because these faculty have worked with the students and have a better sense of their abilities.

    —Continue to refine the process.

    —Increase project linkages with support services since the college already has a comprehensive support service that offers tutoring in any subject a student may request. Address the problem of oversubscription for these support seminars.

    —Develop separate seminars that focus on anxiety reduction and success strategies for chemistry and biology courses.

Figure 1

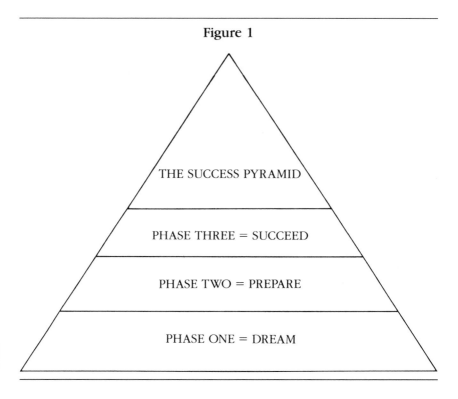

THE SUCCESS PYRAMID

PHASE THREE = SUCCEED

PHASE TWO = PREPARE

PHASE ONE = DREAM

Although several unanticipated problems arose during its first year, this project continues. In fact, two students are now ready to enter the nursing curriculum in 1993 if they remain on track and proceed as outlined. Further refinement of the project has been based on the following lessons learned thus far:

- Students are not always able and ready when the funding is available.
- Capture a student group prior to capturing a coaching group.
- Be prepared to change.
- All lessons are painful, valuable, and important.

Based upon the evaluation, we have redesigned the success program and are looking at a pyramid model. This model has three levels (see Figure 1). Phase one, dream, services large groups of individuals who feel that they can be nurses but are very far from their goal. They need frequent "rah rah" speeches tempered by honest responses about how long it will take. Phase two, prepare, enrolls students in college-level coursework and supports their progress. Students in this phase are linked with their cheerleaders and proceed to learn more about the nursing profession. Phase three, success, supports students who are accepted into the nursing program. These students remain linked to their cheerleaders and are assisted as needed on an individual basis so that they can successfully complete the nursing program.

This refined model will be implemented as the search for success continues.

3

Culture in Curriculum: A Process for Integrating Multicultural Elements into the Nursing Curriculum

Eleanor L. Strang

RECRUITMENT IS NOT ENOUGH

A lmost since the nursing program was established at Central Arizona College, faculty had recognized that Hispanic and Native American students were less likely to enter or to finish the program, and to complete the State Board examination successfully. Faculty recognized their responsibility to help minority students to succeed and tried to do so. Efforts included special courses presented on the nearest Indian reservation, specific remedial attention for less academically prepared students, direct high school recruitment, referrals to counselors, one-on-one tutoring, and other generally accepted methods for improving minority recruitment and persistence.

Over the past few years we have had some success: minority students do come more academically prepared; they have applied and been accepted in greater numbers to the program. In several instances, however, students have not persisted through the Associate

The workshops described were supported in part by a grant from the Arizona Statewide Council on Nursing.

Degree, and the NCLEX-RN success rate has changed less than we wished. In analyzing reasons for this, faculty noted their assumption that minority students must adapt to majority perceptions of health care and education values in order to succeed in the program and in practice after graduation. Faculty wondered whether cultural assumptions in the curriculum might be factors in confusing students, creating conflicts sufficient to deter student progress.

Faculty reviewed their own experiences with students in clinical and advising situations. While one faculty member is an Hispanic woman, the remaining faculty are white, women, and educated in traditional Western nursing ideology. We identified several possible sources for cultural conflicts. We found our minority students were subjected to conflicting values in the curriculum, their socialization into clinical practice, and their relation to the current hierarchy that structures the health care system. Our students also observed minority clients of non-minority nurses and nursing students as experiencing cultural dissonance while in the system.

As a result of these findings, we agreed that a truly effective nursing curriculum for our students and clients required multicultural understanding for both minority and non-minority students. Minority students needed to be able to identify their own cultural dissonance and conflicts in order to judge appropriate responses within the dominant health care system, including the NCLEX-RN examination. Non-minority students, who would be caring for a great many minority clients, needed to see the needs of those clients appropriately within the clients' cultural context. We hope that such changes in perspective might someday eliminate barriers within health education and practice arising from dominant cultural biases.

THE PROCESS

Although to revise the cultural assumptions in an entire curriculum seemed to be a major undertaking, pressures of time and lack of money precluded anything except simplicity. We decided to use a combined workshop and individual review strategy to accomplish our goals. Through a grant from the Arizona Statewide Council on Nursing, we conducted two workshops for faculty using Native American and Hispanic nursing consultants. Value issues, student adaptation problems, and practice situations provided dimensions for future discussion, continued curriculum analysis, and subsequent evaluation of outcomes.

Step 1—The First Workshop

In our first workshop, a Native American Director of Nursing and an Hispanic Nurse Educator shared with faculty their personal stories of nursing education, practice, and patient encounters to illustrate cultural differences from personal perspectives. Participants then broke into small groups. Each group had a Native American and an Hispanic resource person who helped to more specifically identify the values within each culture—Indian, Mexican, and Anglo—that might generate cultural dissonance.

Within the small groups a faculty member, acting as facilitator, guided discussion by using a modified brainstorming technique. Together we produced a list of several concepts from which cultural conflict could arise including: perceptions of self as an individual and within the group, gender and age roles, time relationships, relationships of human beings to the natural world, educational values, death, pain, future and past, etiology of disease and dysfunction, and acceptability of treatment modalities.

Step 2—Individual Faculty Analysis

After this workshop, faculty reviewed the process and the initial outcomes, and recommended changes for the second workshop. They were universally enthusiastic and began to think concretely about changes to be made in the course syllabi and in their own teaching methods. And we began to understand, just a little, how much we had expected from some of our students.

Each faculty member was charged with reviewing her own area of teaching responsibility in order to identify where cultural elements should be integrated and emphasized. This information provided the foundation for the second workshop.

Step 3—The Second Workshop

There was so much new learning at the first workshop that faculty expressed frustration at not being able to hear everything that each consultant resource had said. They also wanted to know and learn our own students' feelings and points of view. Consequently, the second workshop was designed so all could participate in a single group.

This dialog produced a great deal of satisfaction from all participants. We invited Native American and Hispanic students as well as the Native American Director of Nursing and the Hispanic Nurse Counselor who had been resources for the first workshop.

We began the second workshop by considering the student's perspective. Because we teach students to assess before making judgments and performing care actions, we agreed that faculty must also *assess* the student. Some of our students, however, were more aware of their cultural heritage than others. Just as not all Anglos are alike or at the same stage of personal development, not all ethnic minorities are culturally different from the majority of society. Among Hispanics in particular, younger people may be closer to their Anglo peers in behavior and perspective than to those prescribed by cultural heritage. Native Americans, especially if reared off the reservation, may also be less culturally tied to their roots than their parents. We recognized, therefore, that whatever we included in our curricula must be accountable to this range of cultural variation.

In the second workshop, we focused particularly on how the information we gathered would be integrated into the content and teaching process of the nursing program. Recognizing that we must pay attention to attitude building in faculty as well as to assisting students to adjust to the social and cultural value systems in nursing and health care that affect nurse-client relationships, we reviewed performance and cognitive objectives for each module in the successive levels of our curriculum, and noted where cultural information needed to be emphasized or added. Last, we discussed how best to prepare the minority graduate for employment.

Some of what we learned from our associates during the workshop we share with you. However, these findings are not without a cultural context of their own. If their prevailing Anglo-American context excludes aspects significant to our Native American and Hispanic colleagues, then we must apologize for our ignorance.

Step 4—Application of Workshop Outcomes

During the workshop, it became evident that all aspects of the nursing process are affected by the viewpoint of the persons involved and few people fit textbook examples of ethnic identity. As a result, incorporation of cultural information into all aspects of the nursing process—in teaching and learning, in the transition to the professional role, and in adapting to the context in which nursing exists—becomes a necessity.

Assessment. When assessing students, faculty must determine where they are, culturally as well as academically. Students may appear shy or unprepared when they are simply acting as they have been taught in their culture; for example, to show respect and to learn by observing. As teachers, we must not mistake lack of eye contact for dishonesty. Among Hispanics and Native Americans, lack of eye contact is a sign of respect. We must be aware that these same students will rarely offer answers on their own. They need to be asked and given time to respond in their own way. They are not good at asking for help. Within their cultural group, especially among Native Americans, the emphasis is on group relations and the student expects that the group (i.e., faculty and classmates) will know what they need. They must be taught to ask. And above all, faculty must keep in mind that each of the students varies along the continuum between two cultures and not compare one Native American or Hispanic with others.

In the practice arena, assessment in Anglo culture presumes that nurses ask many direct questions, some of which invade personal privacy, and establishes that both client and nurse recognize the dominant power of the nurse over the client. Because it runs counter to their usual social situation, this assumption may generate discomfort in traditional Native Americans or Hispanics. It may be very difficult for a young, female Native American or Hispanic student to be directive to an older person or to a man because of gender and age roles.

Traditional gender roles for Hispanics place the man in authority over women. In addition, Hispanic women tend to be very modest; consequently, they may be reluctant to have male nurses in attendance for gynecological procedures or childbirth. Native Americans, also quite modest, may be more tolerant, allowing the father to be present for birthing, but may also be more comfortable calling a male nurse "doctor." Clinical instructors must assess their students and the clients to whom the students are assigned for such cultural values, and adjust assignments to make the most of clinical interactions. For example, with a large number of male students enrolled, we should rethink how we assign them in family planning clinics, many of which have a high proportion of Hispanic clients.

When learning to assess clients, students may also face the dilemma of finding it difficult to initiate questions related to personal matters such as alcohol consumption, sexual problems, abuse, or other possibly embarrassing topics. Among many Native Americans, for example, respect includes an unstratified social schema in which all persons are equal. It is unsuitable for one to be considered better than another. Consequently, clients will tend to hide embarrassing information. It may be more fruitful here to formulate questions that assume, without judgment, that a person drinks, rather than asking whether that person does or not. Don't ask "Do you drink?", but "When did you have your last drink?"

Students may benefit from demonstration of client assessment by an experienced nurse role model to learn how to be open yet avoid offense. They can be taught to apologize at the beginning as, "I have to ask you something that is important to how we care for you. . . ." Facial expression should be bland and tone of voice respectful. Role playing can help students cope with anxiety before going into the clinical area, with students from different cultural backgrounds providing insight into client responses to other students' efforts. This also contributes to building the student's self-esteem.

Because Native American clients often have difficulty explaining how they feel, it works better to ask them to compare: for example, rather than asking "Are you having much pain?" the nurse should ask "On a scale of 1 to 10, how would you rate your pain?"

ANALYSIS

Analysis always reflects personal values and cultural background. Foremost among these values is the significance of self. Among whites, especially in the United States, the individual is of primary importance. We teach people to have pride in themselves, to be independent, to take care of themselves. Among both Native Americans and Hispanics, the group is paramount. The question they ask when meeting someone will be not "Who are you?" but "Where do you come from?" Self is determined by family, village, or tribal affiliation.

For Hispanics, all family members will want to be present for important events such as graduation. In the hospital, it means that everyone wants to be there when someone is ill. Students must be taught how to set limits respectfully, using the authority in the family group to establish limits on visiting or to reduce congestion in lounge areas. Let that person also speak for the group. The patient may naturally defer to another person, usually an authority figure, in decisions affecting care.

Among Native Americans, tribal beliefs may differ. It will be up to the nurse to determine what approach to take in ascertaining the self-perception of the patient. In either case, the advent of "advance directives" requires that nurses understand who will make decisions for the patient and assure that the appropriate wishes are followed.

Approximately 80 percent of Hispanics are Catholic but many still believe in hexes and in the power of the *curandera* (female healer) or *curandero* (male healer), especially among the older people. Native Americans differ among tribes and some practice mixtures of Christian and traditional religion, particularly when it comes to healing. Students must learn to accept the appropriateness of allowing the *curandera* or *curandero* or other tribal healers and wise persons to assist with Anglo-American medicine. And patients must be allowed to have access to these persons.

In this respect, the Native American Director of Nursing told us of a patient who was diabetic but had quit taking her insulin and following her diet because, on the advice of the curandero, she had been drinking special teas. In some situations she would have been labeled "noncompliant" and perhaps been subject to repeat teaching or written off. Instead, the nurse recognized that she needed to be convinced to *combine* traditional therapy with the Anglo-American medicine to make them both more powerful against the disease.

Hispanic and Native American students and patients may come from situations where life is accepted on a different level than for many whites, and where illness and death or dying carry different meanings. If quality of life may be defined as "whatever makes you happy," for a diabetic Native American this could be eating whatever he or she desires, not going to a clinic, or not having foot ulcers. It may be difficult for the patient to understand that these are not compatible. Moreover, in these cultures, deterioration of bodily functions is as normal as age, and death is accepted as part of the life process. Therefore, loss of a limb may be acceptable and expected.

As Native Americans lose organs to diabetes, they are becoming more likely to consider kidney and corneal donations or blood transfusions. On the other hand, some consider diabetes to be a white man's disease and refuse ownership of it. Their attitude conveys a spirit of "You brought it, you take care of me." Although they may accept dialysis as treatment for ESRD, many prefer transplant. Hispanics, on the other hand, might not think about organ donation because of a cultural belief that separated body parts may be used for sorcery.

We teach Orem's self-care theory in our program. We must now consider modifying our approach to accommodate cultural roles in illness. A Native American or Hispanic in the hospital may consider it the nurse's job to take care of them. When we insist that they participate in self-care, they wonder why they must do the nurses' job and refuse to do their own care. In the sick role they may give over decision making, even the answering of simple questions, to someone else. Thus, when the nurse asks questions, someone else may answer or give the patient permission to answer or tell the nurse that the patient is too sick to do what the nurse has asked. This does not mean that the patient is being dominated against the patient's will. Many patients will participate in some aspects of their own care but not in others. They may be less reluctant to do their own dressings, colostomy, and stump care, for example, than to do injections. Someone else will be expected to do that. This is particularly true for men. Therefore, teaching plans must always involve significant family caregivers.

For many Native Americans, it is more suitable to die at home than in the hospital, and they accept death better than most whites. Requests to be discharged to go to the reservation in the face of impending death should be granted. Care of the body after death varies widely among Indian tribes. By all means ask the family before any action is taken. Some do not embalm, some bury bodies immediately. Some cremate, others consider cremation a sacrilege. Navajos may refuse to touch a dead body. In other tribes, the family must ritually care for or dress the body.

Grieving also varies among tribes. Navajo are not allowed to grieve openly for four days, during which they neither bathe nor wash their hair. Papago will want to see the deceased, regardless of the condition of the body, and often grieve loudly. In any case, wait until the family are finished with their personal needs before sending the body to the morgue and then to the funeral home. Persons who die at home will sometimes remain there for community visitation.

One of the most important sources of cultural conflict for students and clients alike is the concept of time. The dominant culture is time bound. Nowhere is this more evident than in the health care system. Everything is scheduled by day and hour and we document that schedules are met. For Hispanics, however, relationships are more important than time schedules. If one meets a friend, talking to that person is more important than being on time for a clinic appointment.

For Native Americans, time runs differently. Counting by minutes and hours and relating to schedules in the white world must be learned. Faculty must socialize students to punctuality requirements of the course and help students plan.

Native Americans may find it necessary to return to the reservation for obligate tribal responsibilities. Faculty and employers should establish understandings of how much time can be taken and what may be done to make up if acceptable. Students can then be held accountable in the system yet still participate in their tribal obligations. It helps if each student has a support person on the faculty with whom he or she can discuss special needs.

PLANNING AND IMPLEMENTATION

After carefully assessing students, analyzing their needs in their cultural context and our needs as well, we must adjust strategies to accomplish desired outcomes. We are adding some of our new knowledge to the orientation and role content given at the beginning of each term. We will integrate basic Native American and Hispanic differences into each element of the nursing process as it is taught and as it is evaluated in the students' case studies. We found potential for cultural dissonance in many areas of treatment, in client teaching, and in some specific disease entities. We are integrating as much of this information into the content of the course modules as possible. Much remains to be done. However, I would like to share with you part of what we have learned.

Healing need not be restricted to a single cultural approach. Use of the *curandera* or *curandero* or other tribal healer need not conflict with Anglo-American medicine. Hispanic healers lay great store in teas, which are unlikely to have conflicting effects on medically prescribed treatments, medications, or therapeutic diets. Likewise, traditional tribal rituals do not necessarily require suspension of medication prescribed for illness by doctors. In teaching plans, nurses may achieve maximum benefit with integration of traditional with Anglo-American medicine. If the patient believes in it, it is often helpful.

Patient teaching involves cultural implications in addition to those mentioned previously. For example, although Native Americans and Hispanics are gradually losing a traditional reluctance to touch their own bodies, making it easier to teach breast and testicular self-examination, older women avoid mammograms and pap smears. Younger women may accept these procedures more readily.

Boy babies are not circumcised in traditional Hispanic households. This is because circumcision may be considered as torture, or as becoming white or Americanized, or as reducing male virility. Native American babies, on the other hand, may be circumcised on parental request but are not done as a routine.

Hispanics and Native Americans accept common surgical procedures somewhat differently than whites. Traditional Hispanics may insist on specific disposal of body parts, either because of belief in literal rebirth or the threat of sorcery. Native Americans beliefs vary among the tribes as to proper disposal. Therefore, nurses must ascertain the patients' wishes before they go to surgery.

Obstetrics and pediatric nurses will encounter parenting behaviors reflecting values of the person and of the community group. Feeding, dressing or swaddling, parental visitation, and discipline of the child reflect the role of the child in the community and will vary by age, gender, and group. Abortion as a means of birth control is not accepted by either cultural group and if an abortion occurs it is usually kept secret.

Mental health and psychiatric nursing may constitute the most difficult arena in which to differentiate cultural beliefs from aberrant behavior. Hispanics are reluctant to seek psychiatric care for themselves and others, but when necessary are more likely to accept counseling from the opposite gender and different ethnic origin. They would be embarrassed to bring a family member for treatment and would distance themselves. From a treatment standpoint, if clients believe themselves to be the object of sorcery or the evil eye, and express that belief, the nurse from another culture may not understand that they are not necessarily giving evidence of paranoia.

Native Americans in counseling, on the other hand, may want to deal with someone of the same gender and ethnicity. While psychiatric services are often available on the reservation, therapists work more with adolescents. Adults are usually quite sick before they are brought for treatment because it is a sign of respect to deal with bizarre behavior at home and not make it public. Although they are very accepting of psychotic behavior, relatives of Indian clients rarely get involved in family or milieu therapy.

In summary, then, faculty-based learning outcomes include:

- All curriculum aspects, from initial student contact through graduation, within all nursing roles and the nursing process are culturally oriented and interpreted. To complete the nursing program successfully and to pass NCLEX exams, the student from an ethnic minority background must learn to practice in a bicultural manner. To function effectively in a multicultural health care system, students from the dominant culture must likewise understand the minority patient.
- Integration of specific multicultural aspects into the curriculum need not be complicated or a lengthy affair. To accomplish the task faculty must be committed and able to draw upon knowledgeable resources.
- The workshop approach was beneficial to us in several ways:
  —It was fairly simple and did not take a lot of time or money to accomplish,
  —It was locally focused,
  —Those to be affected by change were involved in designing the change, and
  —Having students involved gave them ownership along with faculty.

CONCLUSION

Although we consider our venture successful in integrating multicultural elements into the curriculum, it will be several years before we can evaluate outcomes more rigorously. We do know the process works. Because success depends on the participants and not on the procedure, the method should work in various locales and for any cultural groups, so long as open communication, mutual respect, and commitment to student success are paramount.

4

Caring: A Meaning of
Competence*

Emily T. Slunt

What does it mean to become competent as a nurse? Professional competence is usually defined as ability adequate for a specific purpose or achievement of specific behaviors and outcomes. As nurses and educators, we are expected to measure performance whether this performance occurs in an examination situation or on the job (D'Costa, 1984, p. 28). As Benner (1982) explains it,

> *Carried along by a technological, measurement-oriented age, we have been convinced that many of our problems in nursing education and practice will be solved when we have mastered the current measurement technology available—when we can simply and unequivocally describe the competencies involved in the practice of nursing and measure them. (p. 303)*

I believe that the nature of competence in nursing is considerably more complex than observable, measurable behaviors. Missing in the currently accepted definition is attention to situational demands or

* Reprinted from *Being Called to Care* by Lashley, Neal, Slunt, Berman, & Hultgren by permission of the State University of New York Press © 1993.

context and students' meanings of the nursing experience. How can competence be defined more fully to encompass not only ways of knowing and doing, but also the meanings inherent within a particular context?

EXPANDING THE DEFINITION OF COMPETENCE

For van Manen (1984b), the true significance of competence is what a person "is"—for a nurse, the very being of nursing. Van Manen suggests that how one is present to another is more important than what one does. Competence may incorporate technical skills, but the real significance lies with the meaning of being while doing.

For Heidegger (1962), presencing oneself was contrasted with remaining distant or aloof, being preoccupied with other thoughts even though physically present. Do nurses see competence as grounded in "being together" or "being present" with persons while knowing and doing as a nurse?

The Latin derivation *competere* means "to come together, agree, be suitable." *Competens* builds the definition to include "having the capacity to respond, qualified or adequate" (Webster, 1981). In a root sense, then, becoming competent means "striving together to be sufficient or adequate" (Aoki, 1984, p. 75). Aoki also noted that "competence" as "communal venturing" holds promise for a new awakening of what it means to be competent.

TURNING TOWARD MEANING

In a study to understand meanings of experiences within the context of a clinical setting, I spent time with students enrolled in the second year of an Associate Degree program. We engaged in individual and group dialogue in the clinical setting and met on campus for further dialogue and reflective writing. A research approach to understanding meanings calls for a study of inner world experiences rather than experiences of outer world observation. Hermeneutics and phenomenology have specific importance to research here. According to Hultgren (1982), "The rationality concerned with understanding draws its knowledge [from just such] sources . . ." (p. 4).

Phenomenology is the study of the life world of persons; "the world as we immediately experience it rather than as we conceptualize, categorize, or theorize about it" (van Manen, 1984a, p. 37). Hermeneutics is the analysis of text generated through written forms, dialogue, and action. This mode of inquiry strives for understanding through reflection, analysis, and interpretation of text. In the process, meanings and underlying intentions of persons in particular situations are revealed.

In committing myself to an interpretive study, I chose to shed the comfort and constraint of the technical paradigm, to remove the subject-object dichotomy and an emphasis on prediction and control so as to be free of predefined variables. I adopted a paradigm that required venturing forth to make "a map of meanings" while putting self into the process of the inquiry (Mooney, 1975, p. 184). As Slunt (1988) has put it:

As I looked more deeply with unbounded faith
I found new meanings to hold and entice me
The sense of enclosure is not for one to escape
Rather the hold allows one to grow, to become, to be.

To grow away from the embrace of surrounding arms
Is to move both upwards and outward together
Coming back again to find comfort and warmth
Then once again moving beyond but not untethered.

FOLLOWING A CALL TO CARE

I explored the meaning of the call into nursing with the participants in the study. Together the students and I wondered: What makes it possible for one to be a nurse? What draws people to want to connect with other people, to be with other people, to help other people?

Working with people was grounded into life histories and surfaced through stories told by participants, stories of human interest, stories based in an attraction to people in need and caring relationships. This should not surprise us. "Values of kindliness, concern, caring, and tenderness, generated by art, are buried deep in nursing's consciousness" (Watson, 1981, p. 248).

As this study progressed, I found that being together in a relationship of care paves the road for the journey toward becoming competent. The notion of caring, however, has been distorted as students find themselves called upon to be more than a caring, nurturing helper to patients. Our recent nursing advertisement catches attention with the theme line, "If Caring Were Enough, Anyone Could Be a Nurse." In struggling with our image to the public are we not also struggling with a sense of alienation from the very roots of our calling?

Tensions in following the call surface in the form of two contradictions:

1. Nursing is more than caring and nurturance, but nursing is often not recognized outside the profession for its rich knowledge base.
2. Caring and nurturance are integral parts of nursing, but the curriculum and hospital setting reward theoretical and performance characteristics.

What a dilemma! Can competence in nursing be recognized and valued for reflecting realms of knowing as well as being present together in a caring relationship?

COMPETENCE AS INTEGRATION OF EPISTEMOLOGICAL KNOWING

I explored what it meant to become competent in an epistemological sense. As integration of knowledge occurred, intuitive judgments and actions became possible. Intuitive knowing is gradually achieved through integrating knowledge into one's own personal being as a form of "personal knowing."

In teaching theoretical concepts and skills, we as nurse educators create structures to organize the vast amount of nursing knowledge and to show the relationship between particulars and the whole of an entity. We give our students something "concrete." We describe concrete structures as road maps that tell what you are looking for, where to find it, and how to proceed on the journey toward intuitive or personal knowing.

Becky's description of how she organized an assignment is instructive here:

I have my care plan, my assessment paper, my diagnosis book, my drug book, and my own paper so that I can fill in everything from the report and make a schedule for myself. I make sure I include on it everything I have to do from the nurse's chart, the drugs, the nursing kardex, and new orders so that I don't forget anything.

Tracy's elaboration upon the helpfulness of objectives is also instructive:

Objectives give you something to keep in mind so when you go into the room you don't look like you don't know what you're doing. You feel more confident about something to say. I would feel uncomfortable with myself, I think, if I just walked into the room and started talking to the patient and just stood there and kept going, um, um, and then he or she may think, "Well, what does she know? What is she trying to say?"

Tracy found that the structure of objectives helped her to meet her patient and to bridge the gap in applying theory to a clinical situation. For the novice, self alone is not yet seen as being adequate as a nurse.

Students also come to learn and become competent through practice. Practical knowing or doing, "knowing how," is acquired from experience and leads to clarification, understanding, and the development of theory. As Benner (1982) pointed out, "When a skill is performed in an actual situation, the characteristics of the situation have as much influence on successful performance as does knowledge of procedural steps for performing the task" (p. 304). Seeing a patient with a particular history and illness provides the context and cues. Using the context or patient cues along with the theory moves the student toward competence.

COMPETENCE AS FINDING CONNECTEDNESS

As the learner integrates theoretical and practical knowledge, it is possible to focus on the patient as person and to reflect on the meaning of experiences. We have potential for existential knowing; finding insights, new understandings, and ways of viewing the world, along with epistemological knowing. For Watson (1988), "It is on this capacity of one human being to receive another human being's expression of feeling and to experience those feelings for oneself that the artistic activity of nursing and caring is based" (p. 67).

Practicing the art of nursing calls forth intuition in an existential sense that requires both self-knowledge and knowledge of others. A nurse who is in touch with self, for example, is likely to be more open, more spontaneous, and to have more intuitive insights about patients than a nurse out of touch with self. In this regard, "to see what we are not able to describe in words, much less measure" (Eisner, 1988, p. 20) grows in significance when intuition leads caring to knowledge; for example, knowing what a patient is experiencing within a context of illness.

Even when no treatment is available and no cure is possible, understanding the meaning of the illness for the person and for that person's life is a form of healing, in that such understanding can overcome the sense of alienation, loss of self-understanding, and loss of social integration that accompany illness. (Benner & Wrubel, 1989, p. 9)

In the following story, Mandy, in addition to knowing the prognosis for her patient was poor, was able to reach beyond the physical manifestations of illness to reach her patient as person. She saw him as a person with real life experiences and feelings. Giving the patient permission to disclose allowed growth for both the patient and the nurse.

There is one experience I had with a patient that not only affected me at the time but has left a lasting impression. I was assigned a patient in the IMC with a diagnosis of end-stage COPD and secondary complication of pneumonia. This was a 74-year-old man on a ventilator who was very aware of his condition. He had been hospitalized for several months, and I believe he knew his prognosis was poor. I was assigned to him on the day before Thanksgiving; and, in an attempt to communicate with this man, I remember asking him if he knew what day tomorrow was. He nodded, yes, and clutched my hand. When I further commented that I was sure he had spent many happy Thanksgivings in his life, he began to cry—but then he smiled. I felt in some small way we had established some sense of communication.

In reflecting on this experience, Mandy shared the following:

Being able to connect with the humanness of the patient beneath all the machines and establishing a sense of communication with this patient had a very profound effect on me. I certainly didn't feel competent caring for the technology that was sustaining this man's life, but I did feel competent that I reached and touched him in some way.

Mandy understood the power in the human touch, the power in putting herself in the place of her patient and in anticipating and knowing his unspoken responses during these moments of genuine presence. She did not need a great deal of theoretical knowledge in her background to call up these intuitive insights. They came from within her and all that she brought to nursing in answering a call to care. In reaching and touching another person, Mandy experienced the meaning of a beautiful moment and came to know her own power.

Power within self serves as a source of energy for reaching out to others, for living the call into nursing. More authentic and meaningful encounters become possible. As human beings, we grow through insights, sharing ourselves with others, and learning from others. We find new levels of awareness. We grow and become competent through giving and receiving.

DILEMMAS EXPERIENCED IN BEING WITH PATIENTS

Becoming competent does not evolve without anxiety. Tensions were evident in ongoing dilemmas faced by nursing students, as listed below:

- Students frequently lamented that situations in the hospital setting were so different from those in the campus laboratory and that faculty did not understand. The critical difference, I believe, is finding the patient as a person with feeling, the human dimension within the technical procedures.

- Nursing students may sense a feeling of helplessness when faced with the uncertainty of what to do or say to a patient. For example, what do you say to someone at the end of a lifespan when uncertainty and increasing physical frailty are what we know to expect? Feeling failure to help a person in need may leave one feeling inadequate or vulnerable.

- Students revealed a need to protect themselves. Inflicting pain or watching a patient suffer is in opposition to the "call to care." "In suffering from something we move inwardly away from it, we establish a distance between our personality and this something" (Frankl, 1986, p. 107). Barriers may be built to protect the self-hood of the nurse. Barriers or protective armor can look like care without caring.

- The students see themselves as being in the process of becoming competent but are as yet incompetent. An inner awareness that competence is still a goal to be achieved and never an end in itself leaves both student and teacher feeling vulnerable.

- There is a sense of vulnerability in being responsible for another person, a real person who can be injured. Caring for a real person is not like "selling a hamburger" or "cutting a bolt of fabric." "In the fabric store if you make a mistake you can just roll up the fabric. You cannot do that with a patient" (Berman with Slunt, 1987, p. 8). A person called into nursing is concerned with the value of a life.

CURRICULUM IMPLICATIONS FOR BUILDING NEW MEANINGS OF COMPETENCE

Students expressed a valuing of life and personhood in many ways and searched for a better way of "being" for those in their care. Competence is an evolving process of becoming and growth, a growing spiral, as a person gives of self and receives from others. Anxiety and tension as well as plateaus of comfort and a sense of empowerment are found in this evolving process, but the process continues to spiral again and again toward higher levels of competence. The plateaus allow time for reflection and time for replenishment. It seems as if there is always an inner awareness that competence is a goal to be achieved and never an end in itself.

Meanings of competence include having the knowledge and skill for safe and efficient performance, searching to understand self and other, and intertwining caring with knowing and doing. Competence as knowing and doing is possible through a caring way of being.

What would a nursing curriculum look like that fostered a caring way of being? Could meeting and caring for others be viewed as an awesome experience full of potential and possibility?

Listening for the inner voice is enabling for a caring way of being. Listening is a willingness to understand the self, to meet others, and to let others in—to bring down the walls that too much separate who we are from whom we care for. Telling stories is a way for us to see inside ourselves, to hear the inner voice. Stories also allow others to be part of us as they gain new awareness of our inner way of being. Stories are personal and powerful. Thus, we should encourage students to move beyond a focus on skills to engage in dialogue with their patients, to listen for the inner voice, and to encourage storytelling.

I also find that it is helpful for students to reflect and converse about the meaning of experiences. In the process of reflection, an awareness of the power of self and the strength gained from caring relationships may be appreciated. Also possible are insight and acknowledgment of situation and intuitive knowledge leading to an understanding of the depth and complexity of nursing. Reflection contributes to understanding and also leads to action.

I suggest that students and faculty stand together rather than stand alone. Dialogue for understanding requires being aware of our humanness and meshing as equals rather than power of one over another. Establishing a posture of "being alongside" or "standing with" a student means helping, watching, and supporting rather than "standing over," controlling in a supervisory or hierarchical capacity. "Being alongside" means sharing the responsibility for student learning.

I am suggesting what van Manen (1989) calls tactful speech; an application of thoughtfulness in action, establishing a feeling of connectedness (p. 4). Tact is what makes the good teacher—the teacher who is in tune with the student and knows when to be upfront and when to hold back in conversation. "Tact requires that one knows how a situation is experienced by the other person" (p. 6). Tact recognizes the person and protects what is vulnerable. Tact also heals and enhances self-actualization and growth, strengthening the positive (p. 7). To be tactful together, then, is to comfort and empower, to enhance competence.

Movement toward building curricula wherein ways of knowing and being present to another are consolidated comprise curriculum processes that join persons together in dialogue and reflection. In the process of face-to-face communion, understanding and hopefulness give persons the courage and strength to be free, to become competent in a most comprehensive way of being.

REFERENCES

Aoki, T. (1984). Competence in teaching as instrumental and practical action: A critical analysis. In E. Short (Ed.), *Competence: Inquiries into its meaning and acquisition in educational settings* (pp. 71–79). Lanham, MD: University Press of America.

Benner, P. (1982). Issues in competency-based testing. *Nursing Outlook, 5,* 303–309.

Benner, P., & Wrubel, J. (1989). *The primacy of caring.* Menlo Park, CA: Addison-Wesley.

Berman, L.M., with Slunt, E. (1987, April). *Practical dilemmas relative to teaching caring in the clinical setting.* Paper prepared for presentation at the American Educational Research Association Conference, Washington, DC.

D'Costa, A. (1984). *Ensuring job-related validity of nursing licensing examinations.* Monograph Commissioned by National Council of State Boards of Nursing: Chicago.

Eisner, E. (1988). The primacy of experience and the politics of method. *Educational Researcher, 17*(5), 15–20.

Frankl, V. (1986). *The doctor and the soul.* New York: Vintage Books.

Heidegger, M. (1962). *Being and time.* New York: Harper & Row.

Hultgren, F. (1982). *Reflecting on the meaning of curriculum through a hermeneutic interpretation of student-teaching experience in home economics.* Unpublished doctoral dissertation, The Pennsylvania State University.

Mooney, R. (1975). The researcher himself. In W. Pinar (Ed.), *Curriculum theorizing* (pp. 175–207). Berkeley, CA: McCutchan.

Slunt, E. (1989). *Becoming competent: A phenomenological inquiry into its meaning by nursing students.* Doctoral dissertation, The University of Maryland.

Van Manen, M. (1984a). Practicing phenomenological writing. *Phenomenology + Pedagogy, 2,* 36–67.

Van Manen, M. (1984b). Reflections on teacher competence and pedagogic competence. In E. Short (Ed.), *Competence: Inquiries into its meaning and acquisition in educational settings* (pp. 141–158). Lanham, MD: University Press of America.

Van Manen, M. (1991). *The tact of teaching.* New York: State University of New York Press.

Watson, J. (1981). The lost art of nursing. *Nursing Forum, 20*(3) 244–249.

Watson, J. (1988). *Nursing: Human science and human care.* New York: National League for Nursing.

Webster's new collegiate dictionary. (1981). Springfield, MA: Merriam.

5

Teaching Nursing Content
to the 90s Learner

Jean Simmons

*I*n this chapter, I will present reflections concerning my experience with Suggestive Accelerative Learning Techniques (SALT). The SALT method uses non-traditional styles of content presentation to accelerate theoretical learning. Methods include physical relaxation exercises, mental concentration, and suggestive principles to strengthen the learner's ego and expand memory capabilities. I will describe preparation of self, the room you use, exercises that seem to be best enjoyed by our second-year nursing students, the method of relaxation we use to bring our students "into" today's class, techniques for dramatic delivery of content, the use of "fun and games," and how to achieve a successful passive concert.

My discussion of SALT, the result of a research project that I will also explain, will conclude with pertinent benefits of using SALT, both those we expected and the actual focal and contextual influencing factors that appeared and changed our lives unexpectedly. Because student responses to this methodology are important, I will present them as well. Personal bias or residual influencing factors will be evident in my discussion.

To understand SALT, however, requires that you participate in the process (see Figures 1 and 2). Initially, all that is needed are

47

Figure 1
Salt Plan

Room Preparation
    Chairs in circles
    Posters

Body Relaxation
    Exercise
    Tension waves
    Stretching

Mind Calming
    Magic ball
    Early pleasant learning
    Guided imagery
    Music: Slow meditative or mood

Suggestions
    Learning is fun
    I learn easily

Review Preview
    What we've learned
    What we will learn today
    Why is it important
    What we'll be like when it is mastered

Active Presentation
    Dynamic delivery
    Enthusiasm for the subject
    Your ability in action
    Music: Baroque or classical

Practice
    Games
    Role play
    Work sheets
    Work alone or in groups

Passive Concert
    Summary
    Music: Baroque largo (slow 60 hz.)
    Lights dim

Self-Assessment (Post Test)
    Collect or not choice

Quiet Time

Figure 2

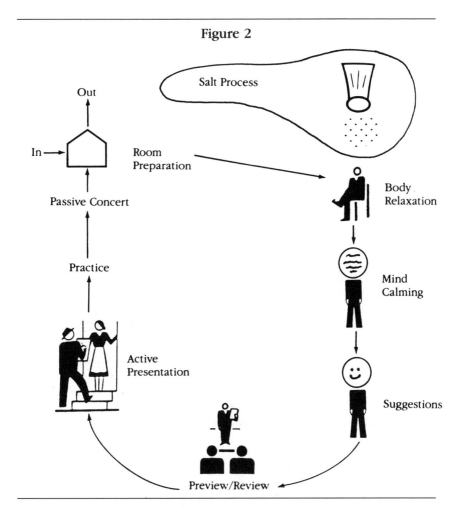

confidence in the instructor and a willingness to explore. Physical relaxation is also necessary; therefore, let's stand and do some arm stretches, side bends, head twists, shoulder rolls, and conclude with a shoulder massage for each other.

After this, please sit, clear your lap, rest your feet flat on the floor, put your hands on your lower abdomen or on your thighs, close your eyes and allow your mind to drift with the suggestions and your body to relax as you listen to the music.

Breathe deeply and evenly, feel your abdomen move in and out, gently let yourself concentrate on your breathing for a moment. Now, concentrate on your right foot, tighten your muscles, hold, and relax. We will continue with a progressive relaxation through the body.

Imagine you are sitting on top of a hill. It's warm outside. The grass has just been cut. You can smell it and you picture the new green. You feel the warmth of the sun on your back. The ground is warm as it totally supports you. You feel a gentle breeze against your skin, caressing you, and you have a sense of inner peace. As you look down the hill, you see a small pond. The surface of the pond is smooth, and you can see the surrounding landscape reflected in the pond. Your body is full of peace. Imagine yourself going down the hillside toward the pond. Feel your body supported and relaxed as you go down. As you get to the edge of the pond, stop and look across the pond and take a deep breath, use all of your senses. Let the thought come to mind of the freshness and newness of the world. Feel the excitement of nature and remember a time in your life when you were learning something you were very excited about. Perhaps it was the first time you rode a bike or went skiing. Bring to mind what it felt like, who was with you, where you were. Bring that special place and that joy and excitement of early learning with you today as we explore some inspiring teaching techniques. Now, shift your position and open your eyes gently—you are happy to be here, alert, and ready to learn. Let me tell you about myself.

I graduated from Greenfield Community College's nursing program in 1965 and returned to teach in 1968–1969. I returned again in 1974 and stayed. My clinical background is in medical-surgical nursing, and I have nursed in Maryland, Florida, California, and Massachusetts. I was taught the basic skills to practice clinically. I was never taught how to teach.

How did you learn to teach? For those "experienced" teachers, do you remember the beginning lectures? For newer teachers, what does "teaching" mean for you? As I prepared to implement SALT, I did a literature review. Included in the history of teaching-learning was a notion of suggestopedia, as expressed by Dr. George Lozanov, a Bulgarian, to suggest accelerated learning and teaching. Dr. Lozanov recognized the power of appropriate suggestion as a critical factor in speeded-up learning (Schuster & Gritton, 1986, p. 12).

In 1986, Schuster and Gritton discussed presenting material dynamically with relaxing music as a way to accelerate learning. For them, SALT makes a broad assumption on an ability to learn. It does not compromise content delivery, it allows for enhancement. The commitment does not require a significant financial investment. The method can be used anywhere. Educators will get to know their students better and vice versa. Students will become more motivated as you, the educator, adopt or adapt all or parts of this educational style.

For 16 years I taught in a rather traditional style. I lectured, encouraged far too little discussion, and covered too much material in too little time, too rapidly. Sound familiar? I have seen a change from the learner of the 1960s to the learner of the 1990s. In earlier years, community college nursing students tended to accept content delivery rather like gospel. Current learners like to be more participative. Our 1990s learner has 40-hour work weeks, three children under 10, is a single parent, 30-odd years old, and participates in community activities. I expect such characteristics are similar for you. Just to see their face in the classroom is a reward!

Content in nursing has become more voluminous, technical, and complicated. In the beginning, I tried to cover everything. I have now come to realize there are at least three, and perhaps even four, different categories of content for the learner: Need To Know, Nice To Know, May Never Be Known—unless the learner puts the pieces together him or herself—and Nuts To Know, a category added by my colleague, Margaret Craig. I have also discovered that I cannot possibly cover everything. Learning is a lifelong adventure. It seems a better use of our little time with our students to initiate a sense of acquiring knowledge that is joyous and positive.

When an alternative teaching style was suggested, one that would focus on the learner holistically, I jumped at the opportunity. I was a little bored with status quo. There is a dynamism to health care delivery, and it was time for me to re-energize my delivery. I do like to have fun, and I was convinced our captive audience was ready also. Finally, I felt a commitment to nursing and the preparation of those who join our profession—they deserve the best we can offer.

I agreed to help a friend, Paul Flandreau, who was shifting gears from surgical practice to the practice of teaching and graduate study. He was convinced there was a better way to teach than "to stuff it in!" Paul acquainted me with previous uses of SALT. Used in many settings, a variety of subject areas, and with several different age groups, SALT encompasses language learning for adults, math for youngsters, and word retention to learning-disabled students, among other content.

IMPLEMENTATION OF SALT

To implement SALT, I first needed to convince my colleague, Arlene Laflamme, to get involved in this project. With her consent, I moved on to our program director, Margaret Craig, and our college president, Kay Sloan. I was aided by timing. Our college community had recently undergone an update of mission and goals. Included was emphasis on exploring and implementing new teaching strategies. Change was welcomed! We forged on.

In the fall of 1988, Paul observed our Nursing 201 classes. He attended two two-hour lectures a week, for 15 weeks. He collected data on test anxiety and examination scores for the semester. In January of 1989, he gave us reading material on SALT. That spring, Paul oriented us to the process. We learned relaxation techniques, practiced "dynamic teaching" to an empty classroom, and reorganized our content delivery for the course materials. The students in our fall 1989 course came to the first class expecting tradition. Arlene and I shared our plan to adopt a different style in teaching Nursing 201 and convinced them they would enjoy our experiments and would indeed find learning not so much of a chore. Fortunately, this group of 50 students allowed us to "pilot" SALT. Our student population included every "personality" type in a normal class. As Paul helped us initiate SALT and gain student trust, he became part of our lives. Although he tried to be a silent observer, there were times we utilized his expertise. In helping us to adapt our voice, mannerism, and dynamism of delivery to SALT requirements, he encouraged us to use "fun and games" that were appropriate for us and our students. Most important, he made us realize we wouldn't fail; with time, our techniques would improve.

By reading this, I assume you are also motivated for change. Learning the SALT technique can be acquired by reading, as we did. Coursework is also available at the University of Iowa. Once you are comfortable with the SALT conceptual framework, you will discern your particular style with SALT in practice.

Arlene and I are very different people. I am linear, a left-brain learner. She is a right-brain learner, visual, and musical. I had to learn about music, imaging, and visualization. She had to deal more with sequence and organization, moving in the classroom, instead of being tied to the podium. As we complete our third year using SALT, we are still adapting the format to our individual styles.

In Schuster and Gritton (1986), SALT concepts were discussed in terms compatible with what I thought teaching should evoke. I am a positive person, and I find I lose myself in my class, once under way. I try to remind the students that our nursing world *is* always *new* because of the ongoing research and technology, but that they likely chose this field of practice because of a fundamental desire to care. I try to foster a respect for them as unique, inquiring individuals. I also encourage questions, as long as students realize that no one can possibly know all answers alone; together, however, we can find them. Because students are receptive learners, they *will* learn in the classroom. While I encourage them to stay with me as much as possible, at times, I also let their minds wander to refresh themselves. By looking at the pictures on the walls, for example, unconscious learning processes can take over.

At the beginning of the semester, we "teach" the concepts behind SALT. I describe to students experiences they might have from adopting SALT. I tell them what their role is and what we, their teachers, will do. We then encourage them to be open and allow themselves to be drawn into the process. I absolutely do not *make* anyone participate, although I ask everyone to consider their colleagues during the quiet times. Actually, I have found the disruptive student eventually calmed by the process.

We prepare illuminations for each class or unit we present. The illuminations give references to the student of particularly significant concepts in the content to be learned. The illuminations, drawn from student textbooks, are figures, drawings, or even special paragraphs that represent the content concisely.

The room environment takes on a holistic approach. Comfortable chairs, useful lighting, restful pictures on the walls and some that are subject-oriented, and an audio system allow for an appropriate preparatory ambience. Arranging the chairs in a circle or in rows for instructor contact/touch with a majority of students is desired. The sound system should allow for microphone voice projection and use of a dual-tape audio player.

The students hear music as they enter the classroom. It is music that lifts them into a learning mode. I use Vangelis' "Chariots of Fire" to inspire them. I begin the class with exercises. Exercise, tension waves, and stretching allow for students to "get ready." They learn to touch one another, difficult for some at first. Later in the semester, hugs happen! A mind-calming segment follows the exercises.

Bringing to mind an early pleasant learning experience and guided imagery prompts students to free their thoughts from as much "garbage" as possible. Not every student is thrilled with this segment of guided relaxation. Some cannot or won't sit quietly. Although you need to allow diversity, you must also control for disruption. It is important, however, to relax the students physically and mentally. You hope to have the student stop worrying about other things and start concentrating on today's class. The student will bring thoughts from this segment of the process into the class over time. I want students to think, "Learning is fun, I can do this, I learn easily, I am ready to learn today." Music for this segment should be slow, or even rhythmless, as with an ocean wave tape.

I begin the actual class with a review/preview segment, associating new material to the context of the entire class curriculum. I try to go back to previous learning to build a foundation for the lecture to be given. For example, with the Gastrointestinal Unit, I will bring back content from the Fundamentals course. I particularly remind students of the words of one of the first-year faculty, for example, who has an unforgettable style of presentation. Using particular phrases or styles of a previous presenter plus putting the content in focus will bring currency to your delivery. I particularly try to emphasize why today's material will be important for students to remember, how useful it will be to know for clinical practice. Often, it is enough to have students recall class content from the previous day. I will then outline the content to be presented, including time sequences, including their break.

I then "teach" the actual class content. Your enthusiasm and mastery of the content will be evident with your delivery. Eye contact, personal touch, when appropriate, and behavior that will draw attention to your teaching of particular salient points are techniques that will draw the student into the learning world. Just as you will be part of the presentation, your student will actively visualize and hear the concepts.

Move about the classroom. Use of visual maps and pictures is effective for a dynamic delivery. Varying voice volume/pitch and tempo will also call attention to change in content. More active participation can be enhanced by music. While I have not used music during medical-surgical nursing content delivery, I have used it during the "fun and games" that follows. Music used should be relatable in some way to class content; for example, using the "Grand Canyon Suite" for a geography class.

"Fun and games" have special places in any classroom, especially those of our highly technical and sophisticated nursing world. It is difficult to let go of lecturing everything to everyone. It took me some time to "see" that learning did occur when an alternative approach was used in the classroom.

In early fall, we like to set the mood of the semester. Arlene and I present our expectations to students, as instructors normally do. In more recent years, we have had our class break into preset clinical groups and set *their* expectations via poster presentations on what nursing meant to them. We discovered mutual goals! Other examples of poster presentations include having students portray the life of a paraplegic while listing appropriate nursing roles. As teachers, we also take part in the class on the stroke patient with students riding in wheelchairs, self-propelling with one arm, breaking eggs with their non-dominant hand, and drawing "dot-to-dot" while looking in a mirror. As Arlene and I wander through the groups, we overhear students discussing what would have been our lecture points. We also have invaluable small-group contact. At the end of the "play time," a spokesperson for the group reports back to the whole class. It is unusual, however, to present a great deal of variety in the poster presentations. Validation of essential content, in a repetitive way, does crystallize the "should know" materials.

Avoiding the usual class "test" is another practice method we have found helpful. In place of the test, we use an overhead projector and flash questions that students answer, then self-grade. Assessment of success is quite evident as you look at students' faces!

Throughout active presentations and alternative learning experiences, we give suggestions that students can easily learn the material, the material is relevant, and the material is interesting to them. We suggest that they will remember the content when it is necessary for them to use it. At the end of class, a passive concert provides a time for review of the class content and a final suggestion that recall will be available at the special time, perhaps in clinical practice or for an examination. The students are thanked for giving their time to me as a faculty person, as well as told to thank themselves for being present. They are encouraged to go out and enjoy the rest of their day. The passive concert is presented using superlearning music, a baroque largo type in the background. The lights are dimmed, and they are asked to get into a comfortable position with their feet flat on the floor, eyes closed, and their hands over their abdomen, feeling the movement of their slow, even breathing. They are asked to hear the music as they hear my words. The summary asks them to picture themselves nursing the type of patient we learned about or perhaps the list of complications of a particular disease. It is a fairly brief highlighting of content. Your words are like an instrument in the musical ensemble; they almost surf on the music, going slow or fast, soft or loud, drawing emphasis to critical content. You read at about the same level as the music or a bit above it. At the end of the concert, I try to settle a minute and let them have time to process the experience. They tend to come to their own summary.

THE DATA COLLECTION

A primary hypothesis here was a probable increase in examination grades as well as a decrease in examination stress.

Paul came to class in the fall of 1988, as an observer and data collector of the comparative (control) group of 40 students. He collected data on self-anxiety with exams by having students take pre- and post-examination pulses and answer a question on their anxiety level. He also collected previous course grades in core nursing courses. At the end of that semester, Paul gave us information on SALT. Previous to assumption of the SALT format, we had six hours of training and reorganized our class material content delivery to accommodate for accelerated learning techniques. Paul returned to our course in the fall of 1989. He observed, collecting data on Arlene's and my teaching technique and self-anxiety on the students at examination time. No relaxation technique was utilized prior to examination, as we felt that would not prepare the students for the reality of the board experience. Students were encouraged to do "whatever they felt would prepare them for each exam." The experimental class had 48 students.

Multiple Analysis of Variance (MANOVA) revealed that the experimental group grades were significantly higher overall ($p < .001$). Exam grades were reported as insignificantly different for exams I and II. However, there was a significant difference for exams III, IV, and V (0.001 to 0.009, univariate F tests).

With the control and experimental groups, the pre- and post-examination self-anxiety scale was not significant. The pulse measurement by group interaction was significant (0.01 level). Experimental group pulses tended to go down more from pre- to post-examination. Control group pulses tended to stay the same (Flandreau, 1990).

Limitations to the study are evident. We used consecutive rather than random classes. As we gained experience with the SALT process, Arlene, I, and our students became more comfortable and confident.

Subjectively, I must share with you the actual experience of a typical class that fall of 1989. In this class, we had the typical passive-aggressives, a free-spirit who seldom, if ever, sat down in class the entire year, students who thought this was a waste of time, and a cadre of those sincerely interested in the process. In time, we observed that all the students were more relaxed, more cohesive as a group, and provided feedback *in* class when they were unable to process content. While we were great with the review/preview, passive concert, and organization, we needed to *work* to use positive messages, physical presence, and have complementary visual presentations. We were now tied a bit to a microphone and it was hard for us to *play*. Arlene and I also began to relax. We found ourselves slower in delivery and not as cluttered in content. Our whole style of teaching began to change as relationships with our students became more personal and human. Although we did not get more personally involved with students than in previous years, we were obviously more approachable. The students' cohesiveness and acceptance of their own individuality was evident. Everyone got to know each other better, a gain for our commuter, community college setting.

The SALT process has changed my perception of the teacher's role. It has also changed learner role expectations. The sense of holism, attention to the student as a very special person, and our reasons for being together for the joy of learning have convinced me there is a better way of doing my thing!

As we conclude, let us return to SALT. Please put your feet flat on the floor, close your eyes, concentrate on your breathing, and the sound of the music. You will hear my voice as *part* of the music, which is a baroque largo style.

Today, you heard my story of teaching, learning, and teaching. You let yourself be drawn into a new process with confidence. Learning to know creates excitement for learning. The way people learn impacts on them holistically, intellectually, emotionally, spiritually. Left-brain learners use language and math logic; right-brain learners use visualization, imagination, spatial manipulation. There is power in combination, and we intentionally appeal to the 1990s learner. The process includes: getting ready, room environment, organized study, music to stimulate and calm, music that would be content appropriate. The student will remember more material, recall it when needed. I shared the results from our research project, the benefits of the initial project for me as a teacher, personal gain, and gain for the student. Consider the future. Schuster and Gritton, suggestive accelerated learning techniques, and SALT bring to mind knowledge and water retention. Physical exercises prepare the learner to sit. Mind calming allows the learner to stop worrying about other things and start concentrating on the lesson for the day. The dramatic presentation allows for imaging, harmonious delivery, and physical presence. The practice phase is an opportunity for fun and games. The passive concert provides music to surf to and time to reconsider the learning time. Let this material pass out of your conscious mind and go into an unconscious space. It *will* be available in a powerful way, when you need it the most! Thank you very much for being with me and sharing your time. After we sit quietly for a moment, we will have time for questions.

REFERENCES

Flandreau (1990). *The use of suggestive-accelerated learning technique in medical-surgical nursing education, a pilot study.* (Unpublished manuscript, Counseling Psychology Program) University of Massachusetts, Amherst, MA.

Lozanov (1978). *Suggestology and outlines of suggestopedia.* New York: Gordon & Breach.

Rose (1985). *Accelerated learning.* New York: Dell.

Schuster & Gritton (1986). *Suggestive accelerative learning techniques.* New York: Gordon & Breach.

PART II

Empowering Students

6

The Curriculum Revolution: Implications for Associate Degree Nursing Education

Mary Beth Hanner
Elizabeth J. Heywood
Marie J. Kaye

*T*he "curriculum revolution" involves a change of focus from a content-driven curriculum to emphasis on collaborative student-teacher relationships, critical thinking, caring, and changing the health care system. This chapter will address the first three foci in relation to Associate Degree Nursing Education. The fourth area, changing the health care system, has been strongly emphasized for baccalaureate nursing students. The intent is to prepare practitioners who can critically analyze the health care system and work for effective change. We believe that it is not realistic to incorporate political activism into Associate Degree curricula. However, Associate Degree nurse educators can serve as role models for students through involvement in professional, political, and community activities that influence changes in the health care system.

There are a variety of reasons why we need to examine the way we teach nursing students in all types of nursing programs. Our health care system is not meeting the needs of our society. Our curricula are overloaded with content that faculty try to keep cramming into courses. Our student population is changing; the students are older, more culturally diverse, and come to us with a wealth of life experiences. Also, the need for caring health professionals has never been more apparent. Proponents of the curriculum revolution are calling for education models that educate rather than train, that are interactive rather than passive, and that emphasize understanding of principles rather than the lockstep execution of procedures.

CHANGING STUDENT-TEACHER RELATIONSHIPS

Empowerment of students through collaborative relationships with faculty is a major tenet of the curriculum revolution. Both classroom and clinical learning environments must foster active learning, nurture assertiveness, and promote interdependent student-teacher roles. A controlling, authoritative approach by the teacher is replaced by a collaborative relationship in which the student and the teacher are partners in learning (Bevis, 1988).

The primary responsibility for learning is placed on the learner. Students can no longer be passive recipients of information; they must actively seek knowledge through the process of raising questions, examining their assumptions, critically reflecting on their actions, and creatively generating solutions to problems. Knowledge acquisition is a complex, multidimensional process that goes far beyond evaluating students' abilities to meet the behavioral objectives listed for a course. In addition to being exposed to content, students truly develop knowledge only when they integrate information into the context of their past experiences, feelings, and cultural beliefs.

CRITICAL THINKING

For our graduates to gain competence in responsive problem solving, curriculum planners are calling for the integration of critical thinking skills at all levels of education. Graduates must be able to critically analyze, define, and explain problems accurately, prioritize, intervene with competence, evaluate the effectiveness of actions, and communicate the results (Miller & Malcolm, 1990). Critical thinking involves learning for understanding, not simply for knowledge acquisition; these are acquired skills, they can be taught and evaluated. Critical thinking is not an optional skill for graduates of any nursing education program. The question is to what extent these skills can be enhanced in the time available to teach both the science and the art of nursing.

Associate Degree nursing educators can foster the development of critical thinking by examining their instructional methods and questioning the educative value of the traditional lecture (Bevis, 1988). Active learning strategies nurture the development of the learner's competency in problem solving and communication. If graduates are to see themselves as knowledgeable, competent nurses, adherence to content "coverage" through a total emphasis on behavioral objectives must be reevaluated. Content coverage is limiting and is increasingly unrealistic in light of the explosive growth of new knowledge and technological changes.

A critical thinking approach encourages the learner to seek and answer relevant questions. One teaching strategy that fosters critical thinking is the case study approach, which can engage the student and the teacher in a collaborative learning process. The teacher can work with the student on the case and can demonstrate effective problem-solving skills through the use of questions in order to identify central issues, and brainstorming to generate alternative approaches to client problems. The teacher, in functioning as an expert learner, can assist in identifying potential value conflicts, as well as the recognition of conflicting perspectives. Role playing can also be used to practice intervention skills such as interviewing, in order to engage the client and mutually seek alternative explanations and solutions for problems. The teacher can and should be involved in the role-playing process and can model how to elicit information that affirms or discredits clinical hypotheses. More advanced problem solving can be facilitated through both case studies and role playing by encouraging students to evaluate supporting evidence, identify errors in reasoning, and differentiate opinions from data-based judgments.

The use of journals is another approach to shifting away from passive learning and integrating critical thinking skills in the curriculum (Hannemann, 1986). For example, journals can be used to improve reading comprehension; students can be asked to list the three most important principles derived from a reading assignment, which then can become the focus of a class discussion. Critical thinking skills can be developed by having students identify what they already know about a subject before they do the reading or engage in the clinical observation. They can also identify questions they have about the topic or experience. Classroom or clinical conference discussion can then be initiated by asking students to share what questions they had before the assignment and what answers they learned. Another helpful purpose of the journal is to assist the novice to personalize or synthesize readings or observations in order to develop a reflective approach to nursing practice.

CARING

Associate Degree nursing educators need to carefully analyze the current literature on caring in nursing, since most of it deals with caring as it relates to the professional nurse. Caring is viewed as being central to, and the essence of, nursing (Benner & Wrubel, 1989; Tanner, 1990). Little emphasis is placed on the graduates of Associate Degree nursing programs. Where does the "technical nurse" fit in? If caring is truly the very core of what nursing is, then the term technical nurse could be considered an oxymoron! We need to look at the message that the term conveys; is there not a better descriptor than "technical" to differentiate levels of nursing practice?

Caring involves such behaviors as active listening, "presencing" (providing full attention to the client, truly being *with* the person, physically and mentally), use of self, sharing of self with another, honesty, and understanding a client's internal frame of reference. Research done on a group of surgical patients indicated that patients categorized caring behaviors into four major areas: good physical care, physical presence, listening to patient fears, and providing patients with information (Cohen, 1987). Don't we expect these behaviors from our Associate Degree graduates? Certainly the universe of caring behaviors encompasses a broad range of competencies based on experience and knowledge. Perhaps we could "level" some of the caring behaviors expected of Associate Degree, baccalaureate, and higher degree nurses in a differentiated practice model. For example, understanding a client's internal frame of reference could involve behaviors that span from an associate degree nursing competency such as "listens to clients to elicit their perspective" to a clinical nurse specialist competency, "demonstrates an in-depth understanding of cultural values and mores and the influence of these on the health beliefs and practices of families and communities." It would be a major challenge, and yet it would help further develop the construct of caring as it applies to expected competency levels for nursing practice.

Tanner (1990) stresses the importance of the culture of the nursing school in teaching caring to our students. If caring is a central value of the nursing program, the culture of the school must support caring between students and faculty. It is often essential to start with faculty development activities that enable faculty to examine their interactions with each other and with students in order to promote more caring practices. Students should be encouraged to care for themselves and their colleagues in addition to caring for clients. Working with expert nurses who demonstrate quality humanistic care provides caring, competent role models who assist in the socialization of the student into the professional role.

An expert mentor could also help the novice learn to provide a holistic approach to client care through the telling of stories that demonstrate vital practice competencies and approaches to complex situations. Expert nurses have many stories, and embedded in these stories are meaningful elements that help to further develop nursing knowledge (Parker, 1990). As Benner has stated, "An enhanced respect for the knowledge embedded in expert practice will set up new agendas for nursing education" (Benner & Wrubel, 1989, p. 402). A case study approach to teaching that uses examples of patients' stories helps students to understand the "lived experience of the illness," the meaning of the illness to the patient. In a practice discipline that focuses on the uniqueness of each individual, case study development and analysis are imperative for theory development (Ruffing-Rahal, 1986).

Another consideration related to caring is the value it receives in assessment of students' clinical competence. Some nursing educators have identified caring behaviors that they include in their performance evaluation tools; students are also required to do a self-evaluation of their caring behaviors (Forsyth, et al., 1989). Other nursing educators call for a balance between evaluating the science of nursing and the art of nursing. Instead of using only quantitative methods of clinical evaluation, we need to legitimize the use of subjective approaches to assessing student performance. Since nursing involves the diagnosis and treatment of human responses, ". . . no one is better able to evaluate students' abilities in this area than the humans who are actually experiencing the responses, the clients themselves" (Curl & Koerner, 1991, p. 24). Evaluation strategies using feedback from both clients and their significant others have been developed to evaluate students' abilities to establish relationships with clients, offer support, provide comfort measures, demonstrate caring behaviors, be organized, keep the client informed, and perform client care adequately. By identifying these behaviors as part of the process of clinical evaluation, we communicate that they are as valued as the technical skills component of the nursing education program.

One challenge that many nurses face is how to effectively blend caring and competence, especially in high-tech settings. The illness acuity level of the patient, the intensity of the acute care environment, the emphasis on cost-effectiveness and nursing productivity, and the increasingly complex patient care technology can act as barriers to caring interactions. A variety of clinical learning environments are needed to help students to learn to provide safe, effective physical care as well as interact with patients in a humanistic manner that indicates the high value placed on the dignity of the patient.

Hospice programs are excellent environments that tend to be more conducive to learning caring behaviors and developing collaborative relationships between students and teachers. The philosophy and focus are obviously on care, rather than cure, and the setting is less physician-dominated than acute care units. Rehabilitation programs and developmental centers can also provide these benefits. Long-term care facilities are clinical learning resources long underutilized by nursing educators. They can also offer freedom from the constraints of acute care settings and allow students to practice with creativity, as well as compassion. As Chopoorian (1990) has put it: "Long-term care is pure nursing. All the work is nursing work: delivery of personal care, developing rehabilitation programs, providing social support to families of residents, dealing with death and dying, assessing and maintaining health, and managing episodic illness" (p. 22).

CONCLUSION

The vast majority of the literature relating to the curriculum revolution deals exclusively with baccalaureate and higher degree programs; the implications for Associate Degree nursing educational programs have not been adequately addressed. Waters (1990) has questioned whether the educational reforms called for are only appropriate for baccalaureate nursing programs: ". . . are those of us in ADN education going to define this as the others' revolution, take up a spectator role and limit participation to an occasional bit of kibitzing? I believe otherwise. The mandate for change, indeed the need for the spirit and energy of change is as compelling for ADN education as for any other program type" (p. 322).

She also stresses the need for discussing all nursing education in a common forum and suggests that we ". . . broaden the framework within which we deliberate education issues to include the whole spectrum of education for nursing practice" (p. 324). If we envision the spectrum of a rainbow, each color is bright and distinct and then gradually blends into the next color, a dynamic whole with discrete components. We need one educational spectrum (or paradigm) for nursing that includes distinctive programs based on educational levels with clearly differentiated outcomes, but part of an interconnected system of nursing education.

We must enter the debate and lend our voices to those who are raising important issues and asking questions that are generated by a new educational paradigm. Nursing claims to be the only profession that is concerned with the whole person, yet we continue to operate, and at times promote, a very fragmented educational system. If the tenets of the "revolution" encompass a student-teacher partnership in the educational process and mutual discovery of new knowledge, shared responsibility for learning, caring behaviors, an egalitarian approach, and a greater value on dialogue, we believe it is essential that nursing educators should work together to incorporate these ideals in all nursing education programs. If the ideas generated by the leaders of the curriculum revolution lead to better program outcomes for baccalaureate nurses, it is imperative that we examine the suggested changes and their implications for our students. Obviously, some of the specific recommendations for baccalaureate programs are not appropriate for Associate Degree nursing curricula; however, the basic approach to the teaching-learning process promotes a shift to more interactive, student-centered models of education. We believe that these elements, as well as caring and critical thinking, are essential for all nursing programs in order to prepare future nurses to meet the health care needs of the twenty-first century.

REFERENCES

Benner, P., & Wrubel, J. (1989). *The primary of caring.* Menlo Park, CA: Addison-Wesley.

Bevis, E.O. (1988). New directions for a new age. *In curriculum revolution: Mandate for change* (pp. 27–52). New York: National League for Nursing.

Chopoorian, T.J. (1990). The two worlds of nursing. *In curriculum revolution: Redefining the student-teacher relationship* (pp. 21–36). New York: National League for Nursing.

Cohen, M.Z. (1987). Caring: The essence of nursing from the patient's perspective. *Proceedings from the international nursing research conference.* Council of Nursing Research, American Nurses Association.

Curl, E.D., & Koerner, D.K. (1991). Evaluating students' esthetic knowing. *Nurse Educator, 16*(6), 23–27.

Forsyth, D., Delaney, C., Maloney, N., Kubesh, D., & Story, D. (1989). Can caring behaviors be taught? *Nursing Outlook, 37*(4), 164–166.

Hannemann, B.K. (1986). Journal writing: A key to promoting critical thinking in nursing students. *Journal of Nursing Education, 25*(5), 213–215.

Miller, M.A., & Malcolm, N.S. (1990). Critical thinking in the nursing curriculum. *Nursing & Health Care, 11*(2), 67–73.

Parker, R.S. (1990). Nurses' stories: The search for a relational ethic of care. *Advances in Nursing Science, 13*(1), 31–40.

Ruffing-Rahal, M.A. (1986). Personal documents and nursing theory development. *Advances in Nursing Science, 8*(3), 50–57.

Saarmann, L., Freitas, L., Rapps, J., & Riegel, B. (1992). The relationship of education to critical thinking ability and values among nurses: Socialization into professional nursing. *Journal of Professional Nursing, 8,* 26–34.

Tanner, C.A. (1990). Caring as a value in nursing education. *Nursing Outlook, 38*(2), 70–72.

Waters, V. (1990). Associate Degree nursing and curriculum revolution II. *Journal of Nursing Education, 29*(7), 322–324.

7

Journal Usage in the Clinical Area: A Guide for Nursing Educators

Claire Ligeikis-Clayton

A n article that recently appeared in the *New York Times* entitled, "Why Johnny Can't Think," faults our current educational systems (curricula) for not making our students think. The message is loud and clear that not only do we as educators fail in developing critical thinking skills that are so vital to individuals and the society at large, but that writing is a critical component in ascertaining these skills.

There is an increasing body of knowledge related to education of our students. As a college professor, I have witnessed a steady decline in the ability of my students to think critically, write expressively, and learn conceptually. This is a concern shared by many of our curriculum theorists as well as researchers who suggest writing as a critical component in all disciplines.

Integration of writing skills, critical thinking, conceptual learning, and concurrent theory with clinical learning are of paramount concern in nursing curricula. The following tool, use of a journal in the clinical area, can be invaluable in acquiring the stated objectives of student learning.

GUIDELINES FOR JOURNAL KEEPING

An important part of our nursing curricula is the clinical component. It is imperative that classroom instruction coincides with clinical learning. Conferencing therefore becomes critical. Objectives of pre-conference include: providing direction for learning days, reinforcing clinical objectives for the day, recognizing the scope and limitations of the nurse's role, and reinforcing "process" learning. Objectives of post-conference include: analyzing the clinical experience, clarifying the relationships between theory and practice, developing generalizations and guidelines in providing nursing care, clarifying thinking and feelings, focusing on patients as people, and reinforcing the learning process (Methaney, 1969).

There are several constraints in our programs that make the above objectives difficult to meet (i.e., lack of conference room availability, not all students actively engage in internal or external dialogue). Based on the stated objectives and constraints of conferencing, this proposal calls for the use of journal writing in the clinical area.

Many studies on the use of expressive writing in education have been made. Some of these findings are listed as follows:

- Expressive writings are crucial for trying out and coming to terms with new ideas (Martin, et al., 1976).
- Skills of writing can help students increase their learning ability, improve communication skills, and enhance cognitive and emotional growth (Fulwiler & Young, 1982).
- Writing is the specific activity that best promotes independent thought (Friere, 1970).
- The goal of curriculum is to develop critical and independent thinking that enables students to make judgments and decisions in a wide variety of life roles and intellectual activities (Sirotnik, 1988).
- Writing allows us to manipulate thought in unique ways because writing makes our thoughts visible and concrete and allows us to interact with and modify them (Emig, 1977).

The proposed journal need not be graded since clinical may be a pass/fail situation and because "free" writing frees the student from the burden of editing and allows the student to become more involved in the discovery process.

Table 1
Rules of Journal Keeping

1. Students should purchase a small notebook at the beginning of each year which they should bring to every clinical for the remainder of the year.

2. The journal should be divided into five sections. Conceptual Writing; Audience Writing; Time Out Writing; Problem-Solving and Self-Evaluation.

3. Journals will not be graded. However, they are part of the students' clinical assignments and must be kept up to date at the discretion of the instructor.

4. Each individual instructor will assign entries and collect entries at his/her discretion.

5. The purpose of the journal is meant to be speculative and written for the benefit of the student, not the instructor.

6. The journal is a means for the instructor to monitor academic growth, personal growth, and patterns of thought.

7. The purpose of journal writing is to improve students' education. It is our goal that through writing, students will be able to develop critical and independent thinking skills that enable them to make judgments and decisions and internalize their experiences in a wide variety of life roles and intellectual activities.

Journal keeping is a means of monitoring academic progress, personal growth, and patterns of thought. Rules of journal keeping are listed in Table 1.

The journal can be divided into the following categories: *Time Out Writing, Conceptual Writing, Audience Writing, Problem-Solving Writing* and *Self-Evaluation.*

Time Out Writing

This writing exercise serves two purposes. First, it can clear the mind and help students make the transition between whatever else is going on in their lives and the start of the clinical experience. At the start of pre-conference, if we can ask them to briefly write what is on their minds, they can vent it and then put it away for the remainder of the experience. The second purpose assumes high stress levels for students during clinical experiences. We may wish to call a time out as a group or individually if we see a great deal of stress. This will help students to regroup or refocus so that they do not put themselves or their patients in jeopardy. Time outs can be called by students as well whenever they feel it necessary. This activity can also be used during conferences if a discussion has become heated, off the track, or if no discussion is occurring at all. For this type of writing you can merely call "Time Out" and have the student write as much as possible for five minutes or you may wish to be more directive with specific questions.

Conceptual Writing

This type of writing can provide valuable insight into the students' grasp of course material. Since our programs are designed so that classroom instruction coincides with clinical learning, it is important that we assess this assumed learning. As instructors, we can pick an area of clinical foci of the classroom courses and have the students relate it to one of their patients for that week. For example, if the focus is infection, we can ask the student to use the content learned in class and correlate it to a specific patient. We may also wish to ask the question, "What did you learn about today—nursing, psychiatric nursing, obstetrical nursing, oncology nursing?" Or we could ask, "What is your definition of an oncology nurse, fluid overload, failure to thrive, mental health?" We can ask students what they are learning in class that week and then give a specific question such as, "In your own words, can you explain cancer cell theory?" These are just several examples that encourage students to engage personally with the course subject matter.

Audience Writing

This type of writing can be used to assist our students in effectively communicating their knowledge not only to other health care professionals, but to clients. By writing for a variety of audiences, we can help our students process knowledge as well as assist them in reality orientation to the profession. Some examples might include:

- "Explain to the physician why you feel this order of Demerol 100 mg. every two hours is not safe."
- "Tell your head nurse why you feel a patient load of twelve patients is unreasonable."

- "Explain to a nineteen-year-old schizophrenic patient why it is important for him to take his medications."
- "Teach a woman in labor how to breathe, push, relax."
- "Explain to a diabetic patient what diabetes is on a cellular level."
- "Teach a four-year-old post-op patient to turn, deep breathe and cough."

These are just several of the many examples that can be used. Hopefully, we can use specific examples from the specialty areas that we are in to further enhance learning. It might be helpful, if time doesn't permit during conference to discuss these writings, to have students exchange audience writing assignments and critically analyze them. Students who share their writing with each other learn to value it more and also become sensitive critics of other people's writing.

Problem-Solving Writing

Students in the nursing discipline must learn to be problem solvers. We will agree there are a multitude of decisions that must be solved by nurses. By giving students hypothetical situations, situations that we ourselves have come across in the past, or situations that arise during the clinical experience, we can help them through the process of problem solving. Several examples might include:

- Make a fictitious patient and staff assignment (or use the current patients and staff on your clinical unit) and have students problem solve staff assignments.
- Have students problem solve either a fictitious or real situation of a confrontation with a staff member, physician, or client.

Another aspect of this technique is called brainstorming where students can write quickly off the top of their heads to generate as many solutions to a problem as possible. Some examples of this technique might include:

- "If I were a head nurse, what could I do to make incentives for my staff?" or
- "How can I involve my staff in continuing education?"

These types of questions not only spark creativity, but aid in the socialization of the role from student nurse to registered nurse.

Self-Evaluation

This type of writing encourages the student to identify strengths and weaknesses and to elicit feelings. Too often, however, we get accounts of how the patient felt or a recapping of the day. We may wish to be more specific and give our students questions such as:

- "How did I feel caring for a terminally ill patient?"
- "How did I feel caring for four patients?"

We may also wish to try some additional creative approaches for self-evaluation such as: have the student comment on the instructor's comments of his or her written work or have the student put himself or herself in a particular role and write a letter:

- "Imagine being a newborn and write a letter to the nurse caring for you."
- "Imagine being a patient at a developmental center and write a poem entitled, 'prisoner of my body.'"

RESEARCH QUESTION

What is the value of using journals in the nursing curriculum?

METHODOLOGY

The 15-item survey (see Appendix A) was administered to 50 freshmen and senior nursing students in different clinical settings. The instructors assigned one journal entry per day, alternating between the four major categories (conceptual, audience, time-out, problem-solving) and an entry in the self-evaluation section each day. The survey was developed based on the objectives of clinical learning, writing, and critical thinking skills. Students completed the surveys anonymously on the last clinical day after reviewing their journal entries in totality. Each item was scored on a 1 (low improvement) to 4 (high improvement) rating scale. As shown in the survey, the descriptors for survey items varied somewhat, but the directionality of items remained constant for all items.

RESULTS

From the 50 students who participated in the project, the overall mean was 38.4 (SD = 10.6). Survey summated rating scores ranged from 18 to 57. Although the sample was small, a coefficient of reliability was calculated using analysis of .93. This indicates that for the students surveyed there was a high degree of internal consistency among the items. The individual item means and standard deviations are provided in Table 2.

Table 2
Itemized Results of Survey

Item	Mean	SD
1	2.354	.785
2	2.583	1.007
3	2.734	.700
4	2.306	1.004
5	2.714	.889
6	2.591	.911
7	2.700	.952
8	2.437	.987
9	2.938	.851
10	2.959	.840
11	2.204	.865
12	2.604	.843
13	2.816	.905
14	2.755	.878
15	2.673	.965

DISCUSSION AND IMPLICATIONS

Based on the individual responses of the questionnaire, we can see the majority of the questions were rated at 2.5 or higher by the students. We can conclude, then, that the students felt a significant improvement in their development of clinical objectives, conceptual learning, concurrent theory with practice, writing, and thinking skills.

Of particular interest were questions nine and ten which had the highest means. Question nine related the extent the journal aided in getting in touch with feelings. Question ten addressed the journal aiding in analyzing/reflecting on the clinical experience. The ability to identify feelings and analyze the clinical experience is of primary importance in our curriculums. Question fifteen addressed the overall benefit of the journal to the students, which demonstrated the usage of journals being of significant benefit to them.

It was also interesting to read some of the descriptive responses which included:

- "The journal was a place where I could express my thoughts and feelings without limits."
- "My journal is an exact reflection of me."
- "I found the journal to be useful and thought-provoking."
- "The journal is a good way to finalize the end of a clinical day."

I also found, on several occasions, students asked me for their journal entries with eagerness and one student in the group used her journal at her place of employment and personal areas in her life.

CONCLUSION

The above results, statistically and descriptively, coupled with the objectives of writing skills, critical thinking skills, conceptual learning, and concurrent theory with clinical learning, reflect the effectiveness of journal usage in our nursing curricula. The purpose of journal writing is to improve students' education. As educators, we can enhance our students' learning through journal writing. It is our goal that through this writing students will be able to develop critical thinking skills that enable them to make judgments and decisions while internalizing their experiences in a wide variety of life roles.

REFERENCES

Emig, J. (1977). "Writing as a mode of learning." *College Composition and Communication* 28:122–128.
Friere, P. (1970). *Pedagogy of the oppressed.* New York: Herder and Herder.

Fuller, T. and Young, A. (1982). *Language connections: Writing and reading across the curriculum*. Urbana, IL: National Council of Teachers of English.

Martin, N., D'Arcy, P., et al. (1976). *Writing and learning across the curriculum*. London: Ward Lock Educational.

Methaney, R. (1969). "Pre and post conferences for students." *American Journal of Nursing* 60:286–289.

Sirotnik, K. (1988). "What goes on in classroom? Is this the way we want it?" in Meyer and Apple (eds.), *The Curriculum*. New York: State University of New York Press.

APPENDIX A

Date: _____

Name: (Optional) _____

Evaluation of Journal Usage in Clinical Nursing

INSTRUCTIONS: Please circle the response that best answers the question.

1. Did the journal improve your skill in expressing yourself?

   Not improved
   Somewhat improved
   Moderately improved
   Improved a great deal

2. How would you judge the use of a journal in assisting you to clarify the relationship between theory (classroom) and practice (clinical)?

   Did not assist at all
   Assisted somewhat
   Moderately assisted
   Assisted a great deal

3. How would you rate the use of a journal in assisting you with your problem/solving abilities?

   Poor
   Fair
   Good
   Excellent

4. To what extent did the journal improve your communication skills with various audiences? (patients, doctors, RN's)

>Not improved
>Somewhat improved
>Moderately improved
>Improved a great deal

5. Did the use of a journal aid you in critically analyzing yourself (self-evaluation)?

>Did not aid at all
>Aided somewhat
>Moderately aided
>Aided a great deal

6. To what extent did the journal assist you in being more personally involved with clinical?

>Did not assist at all
>Assisted somewhat
>Moderately assisted
>Assisted a great deal

7. To what extent did the journal enhance your independent thinking skills?

>Did not enhance at all
>Enhanced somewhat
>Moderately enhanced
>Enhanced a great deal

8. How would you judge the use of a journal in assisting you to develop guidelines and generalizations in providing nursing care?

>Did not assist at all
>Assisted somewhat
>Moderately assisted
>Assisted a great deal

9. To what extent did the use of a journal aid you in getting in touch with your feelings?

>No extent
>Small extent
>Moderate extent
>Large extent

10. Did the journal aid you in analyzing/reflecting on the clinical experience?

> Did not aid at all
> Aided somewhat
> Moderately aided
> Aided a great deal

11. Do you feel the use of a journal has increased your knowledge base?

> Did not increase at all
> Increased somewhat
> Moderately increased
> Increased a great deal

12. How would you evaluate the use of the journal in assisting you to focus on patients as people?

> Did not assist at all
> Assisted somewhat
> Moderately assisted
> Assisted a great deal

13. How would you rate the use of a journal in aiding you to explore your own values/morals?

> Did not aid at all
> Aided somewhat
> Moderately aided
> Aided a great deal

14. To what extent did the journal assist you in reality orientation to the profession of nursing?

> Did not assist at all
> Assisted somewhat
> Moderately assisted
> Assisted a great deal

15. To what extent was the journal of benefit to you?

> No benefit
> Some benefit
> Moderate benefit
> Great benefit

Additional Comments:

8

Partnership for Change: Improving the Medication Experience

Mary Jo Boyer
Carol Lillis

THE PHILOSOPHY OF TOTAL QUALITY MANAGEMENT

*I*n this chapter, we will share the results of a successful partnership among students, faculty, and practicing RNs, a partnership that has resulted in change. That change is reflected in the way faculty and students work together to implement new ways of learning, ways most often suggested by our students. Another change that resulted from our partnership was the way new graduates perceive their competence and confidence in giving patient care. Change was also seen in the way hospital administrators view our graduates who now come to them empowered to accept the challenges of continuously improving the delivery of care; in the way we, as educators, proactively engage our students and ask them "How can we improve the quality of the product we are delivering to you, your education?", and in the way we view our students as our *"customers."*

Although it is difficult to conceptualize this perspective of *customer*—it has taken me four years to feel comfortable with the term—and some will prefer to use the term *consumer*. Whatever term you use, the focus is still the same.

Who, then, are our customers? Our customers are our patients, students, faculty, and clinical affiliates. When do we use total quality improvement (TQI)? We use it when a customer is dissatisfied with the quality of a service, when change is necessary, when you need information about a system from those directly involved in the system, and when you need to evaluate whether quality was delivered.

The framework supporting this system of collaboration, empowerment, and improved quality patient care is total quality management (TQM) or total quality improvement (TQI). Total quality management is an evolutionary (and in some sectors, a revolutionary) paradigm shift in organizational management philosophy and process that challenges the traditional, hierarchical management styles of the last several decades. Total quality management (TQM) embraces organization-wide teamwork and commitment that strives for continuous process improvement based on data-driven decisions (statistical quality control) that result in the delivery of quality services and products that exceed the consumer/customer's expectations.

The stimulus for the total quality management evolution began with industry and business in the 1980s when it became apparent that "poor quality" was causing businesses to lose billions of dollars a year. Some corporations accepted the challenge for survival by adopting Dr. W. Edwards Deming's philosophy and principles of total quality management. In concert with this movement, the Joint Commission on Accreditation of Healthcare Organizations issued its "Agenda for Change" in 1990. At the same time, higher education in nursing was calling for a curricular revolution away from the traditional Tylerian model to a more egalitarian approach supportive of collaboration and empowerment.

Although TQM is participatory and collaborative, it is *difficult* to institute and use consistently. It is not easy, for example, for managers who have traditionally been rewarded and promoted for effecting change through autonomous decision making (the benevolent dictator model) to encourage and live with team decisions and consensus. Total quality management is a process that should involve everyone, however, use data for decision making, focus on quality and the customer, empower participants to effect change by involving them in the process, and focus on continuous improvement.

As a management framework and in these fiscally conservative times when nursing education is challenged to do "more and better" with less money, less support resources, less faculty, and less time, use of TQM becomes paramount. Such use also involves engaging our students in helping us improve how we educate them.

It is important to remember that the medication administration pilot project that we will describe exemplifies the TQI process. But it is only a piece of the pie. The larger perspective concerns student, faculty, and hospital staff involvement in curricular change; total commitment to the delivery of quality nursing education (as defined by internal and external customers); empowerment of our students and graduates through knowledge and experience with data-driven decision making; and support of our nurses as they become change agents in the health care arena and improve the quality of patient care.

We chose a project that the students identified as high priority and involved everyone connected with the process: students, faculty, and affiliating agencies. The purpose of the project was clear—to improve the student's medication experience—and our data show success in this effort. We wanted the improvement to be a collaborative effort with all the participants empowered to effect change, and we were able to do this by using Total Quality tools and techniques that rely on data-driven improvement.

Most of all, we wanted to improve patient care by educating nurses who can effect change by using data. Traditionally, nurses have been viewed as powerless players in a health care system that devalues their opinion and worth. Nurses "burn out" trying to deliver quality care in settings where decisions about their working conditions are made by those only remotely aware of what it's like to be a nurse. TQI is a structure for nurses to use data and effect change through a unified voice.

We will now share an example of how we used TQI tools to change how we teach medication administration. Our intent here is not to prescribe a certain form or to ask for replication of our research study, but to describe an example of a partnership that works.

THE MEDICATION ADMINISTRATION PROJECT

Listening to Our Customers

Our discussion of an alternate method of medication administration centers about a demonstration of TQI principles and techniques in action with involvement of all partners.

Initially, the impetus to change medication administration came from students. In informal conversations with faculty, second-year students expressed the need for an expanded medication experience to better prepare them for their practice as staff nurses. Similar statements were consistently recorded on end-of-year program and course evaluations by a number of students at various levels in the nursing program. As we listened to our customers, the students, the need for an alternate delivery system became even more apparent.

Faculty expressed a willingness to change but wanted to see some data that indicated the need for a change. Statements like "We've always done it this way" or "Let's not reinvent the wheel" were voiced but a commitment for change still existed if the data suggested that a different approach would be beneficial to students.

Clinical agencies, when surveyed informally at affiliate meetings, indicated they needed a graduate who can give multiple medications to a more acutely ill patient. One agency expressed concerns about confusion and errors occurring when we care for certain patients but don't necessarily administer medications to each and every one of those patients we have selected for care.

Using Data for Decision Making

The current medication experience consists of three days of medication administration without a patient care assignment followed by patient care experiences without any additional medication administration. Survey data collected from second-year students about their first-year medication experience indicated the following:

- 68 percent gave 10 or less oral medications
- 88 percent gave less than 4 IM injections
- 85 percent gave less than 4 SQ injections

The current medication administration process was reviewed for consistency and to identify areas of complexity. A flow chart and fishbone diagram (Figure 1) indicated several problematic areas where change was appropriate—particularly in the area of "number of medications given."

Figure 1
Flow Chart/Fishbone Diagram

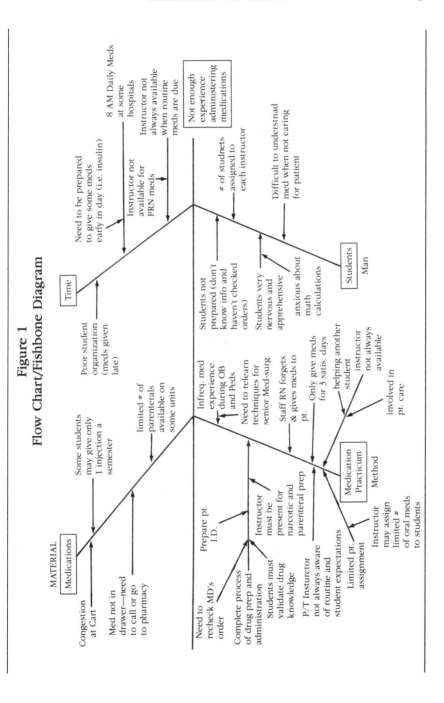

Beginning the Improvement Process

After reviewing the data, faculty discussed various suggestions for improving the experience. Concern for safety was paramount. Based on collaboration with the students and input from our agencies, faculty decided to improve the medication experience. This participatory partnership resulted in a mutual decision to expand the number of medication opportunities for each student. A pilot group of students (24 students—3 groups of 8) who were freshmen and due to begin their medication experience was selected.

A focus group was formed out of the students in the pilot group with faculty responsible for clinical supervision. Several agency representatives also collaborated on an Improvement Statement. This latter group of representatives agreed to improving the students' competence and confidence in medication administration and to reducing their *anxiety.* Operational definitions, as listed below, were clarified for consistency:

- *Competence:* Giving the correct medication (including dosage and route) to the correct patient at the right time.
- *Confidence:* Self-assurance.
- *Medication Administration:* Giving medications by way of multiple routes to assigned patients.
- *Anxiety:* Apprehension or uneasiness related to the administration of medications.

To improve competence, the medication experience was changed from the traditional method (three students at one time giving medications for three satisfactory days with the remainder of the clinical days consisting of patient care only) to a more focused experience. All eight students gave medications at the same time (a functional experience with no patient care involved) for three days followed by patient care with medications included for the remainder of the clinical days. The faculty involved all commented on their increased stress as they struggled to safely control this enlarged experience. Students were delighted with the number of medication opportunities while faculty noted their own anxiety levels increasing.

To measure anxiety and the expectation of increased confidence at the end of the experience, Speilberger's State-Trait Self-Evaluation Questionnaire was administered. Before clinicals began, all students (the 24 students in the pilot group and the remainder of the students comprising the control group) completed the "Trait" section of the questionnaire and completed the "State" section prior to and after the medication experience was completed.

Collecting the Data

As we collected data, we expanded the partnership to include another internal partner—our research department—that assisted us by analyzing our data. We collected information on the number of medications given by the pilot group as well as the control group and observed the results listed in Table 1.

The students in the pilot group were particularly pleased with the results as well as with the fact that they had input and played a role in the change process. Interestingly, we observed the Hawthorne effect with other faculty as they attempted to secure as many medication opportunities as possible for their students in the control groups during their limited three-day experience.

Data collection continued when this first pilot group moved into their Senior Medical-Surgical experience after this initial semester of medication administration experiences. Senior level faculty were unaware of which students had been in this experience group (blind study) and used a simple survey tool to rate all the students at the end of the semester on their medication skills. When the original pilot and control groups were compared, results were not statistically significant. Factors that may have influenced these results include the fact that all scores were combined and one of the questions referred to IV medications that the students do not complete until their senior-year experience. One recommendation for next year may be to look

	Table 1	
	Pilot Mean	Control Mean
Medications PO	33.6	18.3
IM	2.2	.95
SQ	5.6	1.9
Other	6.8	1.9

at each score separately to see whether certain area or skills are indeed significant.

This first pilot group was surveyed after NCLEX scores were received and RN licensures granted. One of the original 24 students did not pass the NCLEX examination and was eliminated from the data collection group. A color-coded survey tool was used (pink-pilot; blue-control) and a stamped, addressed return envelope was included. Eighty percent of the surveys were returned and many included lengthy comments with suggestions for improvement in other areas of the nursing program. Many former students expressed appreciation for being included in this experimental experience with other feedback positive. The percent of entry-level RNs who rated their competence with medication administration as "excellent" was higher for oral, SQ, and IV routes of administration for those in the pilot group. Scores were similar for both groups for the IM route. Sixty-nine percent of the pilot group rated their confidence level when giving medications as "excellent" while 53 percent of the control group did the same.

Results of the State-Trait Anxiety Tests were tallied by our researcher and this original pilot group had a significant decrease in anxiety at the end of this first medication experience when compared with the scores of the control student group.

One final piece of data collection will be to re-survey this original group six months into practice. We plan to invite the pilot group and an immediate supervisor to campus for a dinner meeting to assist us in determining or assessing qualitative issues. In an effort to continue improving this experience, we plan to ask participants in the group "What else can we do to improve the medication experience?"

Collaborating on Future Changes

After the initial experience with the pilot group, all partners agreed on several changes for the next group. The selection process was randomized by selecting every third student, the pilot group was enlarged to include 35 students, and the process was changed slightly. Four students at one time, instead of all eight, administer medications for three satisfactory days while the other four students deliver patient care only. After the intense medication experience is completed, students give patient care and medications to all their patients.

CONCLUSION

In conclusion, this total quality improvement project is an effective example of these following principles in action:

- Involve everyone.
- Focus on the quality of the experience.
- Use data continuously throughout the process.
- Empower participants to effect change.
- Continuously improve.

9

A Unique Approach to First Semester

Jean Flood
Lynn Schneider

CURRICULUM HISTORY

*A*s a result of changing health care needs in the community, the Associate Degree Nursing Program at North Central Technical College (NTC) in Wausau, Wisconsin, implemented a revised curriculum in fall 1990. The Roy Adaptation Model of Nursing provides the basis for conceptualization of the nursing process. The individual courses are organized along the wellness/illness continuum. Faculty members have revised teaching methods to incorporate newer concepts of critical thinking.

Future Community and Nursing Needs

To ensure that the new curriculum would meet both current and future needs of our community and our graduates, we sought information from a variety of sources. The faculty reviewed nursing and health care literature to obtain material about national and regional trends in nursing. The recommendations and criteria for nursing education from the National League for Nursing (NLN), VTAE, and

Wisconsin Board of Nursing were considered. Our advisory committee, consisting of representatives of area health care agencies and NTC graduates and students, provided information about the qualities of nurses that were needed in our immediate district. The committee delineated the strengths and weaknesses of our program graduates and predicted their future needs. Not surprisingly, the information from these various sources was consistent and reflected what our faculty had identified as areas of importance, including: critical thinking, gerontology, health care needs of the non-hospitalized individual, communication skills, concepts rather than content, and nursing theory.

Our advisory committee emphasized that our graduates needed to develop critical thinking skills. Psychomotor skills could be refined during new employee inservice, but critical thinking could not. In addition, we needed a nurse theorist to build our curriculum.

Conceptual Model

After selecting the Roy Adaptation Model of Nursing as a valid framework for the curriculum, the next logical step in the curriculum development process was to create a conceptual model to illustrate the philosophy of the nursing program. The model needed to fulfill three criteria: to define faculty beliefs about person, environment, health and nursing; to be easily understood by our Associate Degree Nursing (ADN) students; and to be reflective of the Northcentral Wisconsin area that the college serves. The faculty concurred that "the tree" could visually depict both the paradigms of nursing and the major components of the curriculum.

The NTC nursing faculty believe that each person is a unique bio-psychosocial/spiritual being who is in constant interaction with the environment. The tree symbolizes this individualism (Figure 1). Each tree has its own unique characteristics. As these characteristics develop, the tree continuously interacts with its internal and external environment. Both the internal and external environment continually exert effects on the person. Likewise, the tree responds to ever-changing external stimuli and adapts to the influence of its internal environment.

The faculty believe that health is the result of adaptive behaviors acceptable to the individual. Each person has the right to health information so informed choices can be made. The tree, in its

Figure 1

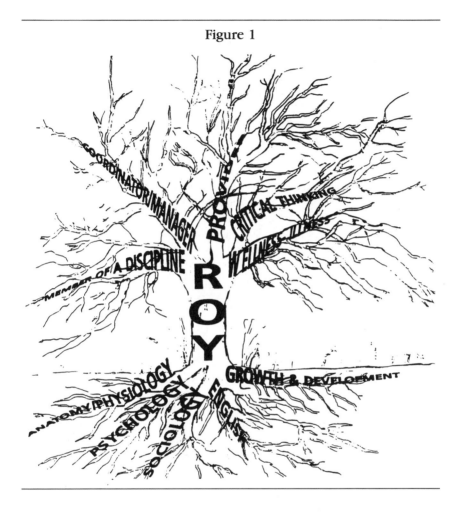

uniqueness, chooses a level of adaptation consistent with the summation of the environmental influences. Each tree grows to its fullest potential as it adapts externally to the multiple stimuli of nature and to the necessary modifications of the internal environment.

Nursing is a multifaceted discipline that uses interpersonal skills to assist persons in adapting across the lifespan. The entire tree thus symbolizes nursing's ability to utilize interpersonal interaction infused with the Roy Adaptation Nursing Process to promote adaptation. The overlapping of the branches, for example, demonstrates nursing's multiple roles and skills used to assist persons as they choose a level of health.

The tree also visually demonstrates the components of NTC's Associate Degree Nursing curriculum. The focus of the nursing program is the student. As adult learners, each student brings a uniqueness based upon previous learning and life experiences. The soil represents this diversity of students and acknowledges the distinctive characteristics they bring to the nursing program.

The roots of the tree exemplify the base that the nursing curriculum is built on. The tree's hidden root system is as expansive and interrelated as the visible branches. Students are required to take courses in anatomy, physiology, English, sociology, growth and development, and psychology. These courses provide a secure foundation for the nursing courses.

Roy's Adaptation Model of Nursing is visualized as the trunk of the tree. Roy's model provides a framework for students' conceptualization of the nursing process.

Five equal branches represent the five threads of the curriculum. Three of these threads—Provider of Care, Coordinator/Manager of Care, and Member of a Discipline—were identified as roles of the Associate Degree nurse by the NLN. The fourth thread of the curriculum is Critical Thinking. To create nurses who are competent decision makers, the faculty felt strongly that the student be charged with the responsibility of learning to think in a critical manner. The final thread, Wellness/Illness, provides the curriculum with the logical sequencing of courses.

Nursing Program Courses

The first semester, Supporting Adaptation in Health, emphasizes the nurses' role in the promotion and maintenance of wellness in persons throughout the lifespan. Students are involved in two clinical rotations. For six weeks, students concentrate on healthy mothers and infants and explore the family as it adapts to new roles. The second rotation, Primary Care, is addressed later in the article.

Second semester, Rehabilitative Adaptation in Health, focuses on the use of the Roy Adaptation Model as the basis for practice with adults who are expressing ineffective responses to acute situations.

Clinical sites utilized are the acute surgical unit and extended care settings.

During the third semester, Rehabilitative Adaptation to Health, the students focus on persons with ineffective responses to chronic and/or multiple situations. Medical and acute psychiatric clinical units provide the students the opportunity to apply complex concepts.

The final semester, Integrating Adaptation Concepts, requires the student to evaluate and synthesize new and previously learned knowledge to care for persons across the lifespan. The Home Care setting provides the challenge necessary to internalize many concepts and integrate management of focal and contextual stimuli. Integration of the Provider of Care, Coordinator/Manager of Care, and Member of a Discipline roles are synthesized during a seven-week management rotation. The final experience, Role Transition, is a 64-hour preceptorship in a clinical area chosen by students. The five terminal program outcomes reflect the program threads and are used to measure student achievement during this rotation. Students create their own learning objectives from the program outcomes and measure daily progress through journal entries and conferences with their nurse preceptor.

PRIMARY CARE ROTATION

Our first semester was developed to help students focus on wellness and begin to think critically. Students spend six weeks in the primary care rotation. Clinical objectives are designed by the students. Each week the students focus on communication skills, wellness, self-direction, and self-assessment. Weekly topics include teaching skills, cultural influences on health, and health needs of the elderly.

Clinical experiences are designed around Knowles' (1984) assumptions regarding the adult learner. Knowles believes that students are internally motivated by their desire for a better quality of life, greater self-confidence, and greater self-actualization. Adults are self-directed although initially many want to be told what to do. Early sessions in the first clinical are generally spent helping the student develop self-direction. Rather than telling students what to do, faculty guide students in designing their own weekly learning experiences.

According to Knowles (1984), adult learners are ready to learn when they experience the need to learn. At times it may be necessary for the faculty to help the students see their needs. This is accomplished in the primary care rotation through interactions with the faculty, clients, and other health professionals that help the students identify gaps between what they know now and what they will need to know as professional nurses.

The faculty believe students' past experiences are an important part of who they are—to ignore these experiences would be to ignore the student. The primary care rotation seeks to utilize the rich and diverse past experiences our students bring with them. Individualized learning plans adapt to each student's level of knowledge. During weekly conferences with the entire clinical group, students share their diverse experiences and learn from each other.

Knowles' final assumption is that the adult's orientation to learning is centered on a desire to perform a task, solve a problem, or live in a more satisfying way. The primary care clinical rotation is designed to reflect the health care needs in each student's community and social group to promote immediate application to their life situation. When students plan clinical experiences within their own communities, faculty travel to these locations to facilitate the process. These assumptions are summarized in Table 1.

Our experiences in the last four semesters with the primary care rotation have been remarkable. After initial hesitation, students have

Table 1
Application of Assumptions of Adult Learners

	Assumptions	Application
Concept of Learner	Self directing	Identify own learning needs
Role of Learner's Experience	Rich and diverse, students are resources for each other	Individualized learning plans, sharing in weekly conferences
Readiness to Learn	Determined by the need to know	Interactions with faculty, health professionals and clients
Orientation to Learning	Centered on life, task or problem	Experiences developed for people they meet everyday in their lives
Motivation to Learn	Internally motivated	Learner designed activities

responded positively. Student experiences have been diverse, including: conducting a health fair; safety assessments in the homes of elderly people; health promotion classes at local clubs, industries, and schools; nutrition and meal preparation classes with families; and developing interviewing techniques with a variety of people. Most students have expressed a better understanding of the elderly and breakdown of preconceived ideas.

The clinical experiences have been rewarding. They have provided a sound foundation for the student to grow throughout the rest of the program.

REFERENCES

Knowles, M. S. (1984). *Androgogy in action*. San Francisco: Jossey-Bass.
Roy, S. C., & Andrews, H. A. (1991). *The Roy adaptation model*. Norwalk, CT: Appleton & Lange.

PART III

Responding to Change in Health Care Delivery

10

Community Health Concepts in Associate Degree Curriculum

Roberta Hunt
Ellie Slette
Mary McKee

*I*n this chapter, we will describe the need for including community health content in the preparation of Associate Degree Nurses (ADNs). For those who might wish to consider a similar curriculum revision, we will also trace the development of the course.

Inver Hills and Lakewood Community Colleges provide a two-year Associate Degree Nursing Program that began graduating students in 1975. This joint program offers a complete curriculum at both Inver Hills Community College, located in Inver Grove Heights, and Lakewood Community College, located in White Bear Lake. Each of the colleges has a student population of approximately 2,000 students with each campus graduating 70 to 80 nursing students every year. The program includes both a basic and accelerated track with the latter providing advanced placement for licensed practical nurses (LPNs).

The fall 1991 student profile of the nursing students in this program reflected more than 80 percent over the age of 26; 70 percent are parents, with 27 percent of this group single parents; 9.2 percent are men, and 5 percent are African Americans.

The Nurse in the Community is a two-credit required course offered twice every academic year, in the fall and spring, for the accelerated students and the basic students respectively.

In 1983, another course, "The Nurse and the Community," was planned and introduced into the curriculum of the Inver Hills-Lakewood Associate Degree Nursing Program in St. Paul, Minnesota. Admittedly, the course title may cause a visceral reaction in nurse educators who are currently grappling with definitions of scopes of practice for the projected two levels of nursing. The course design, however, reflects one faculty's efforts to provide students with the knowledge base and skill-development needed in today's marketplace where early discharge of seriously ill clients is dictating significant changes in nursing practice.

Traditionally, ADN programs have included selected community health concepts such as referral to community agencies and health team collaboration. However, these concepts have been interspersed throughout the curriculum and not organized into a distinct course with objectives that emphasize "continuity of care" within the scope of Associated Degree nursing practice.

The Inver Hills-Lakewood faculty have struggled to identify the legitimate parameters of course content and expected learning outcomes while maintaining the integrity of the ADN scope of practice. The notion that Associate Degree nursing curricula should include a full-blown community health nursing course that would prepare graduates for certification or practice in public health nursing was deemed inappropriate and was never proposed or considered.

NEED FOR THE COURSE

Health care has undergone rapid and significant evolution in the past few years and nursing practice itself reflects this continuing state of transition. As federally mandated changes in reimbursement for health care services were about to be implemented in 1982, faculty of the Inver Hills-Lakewood nursing program were concerned that the care of hospitalized patients would soon require different and expanded knowledge and skills from ADN graduates.

Average length of stay of hospitalized patients was expected to decrease significantly; thus, the typical patient would be more acutely ill. The faculty anticipated that the hospitalized population would require increasingly more sophisticated levels of nursing care and that patients would be discharged in increasingly more debilitated states. Furthermore, patients anticipating discharge from the hospital would have greater need for comprehensive discharge planning and referrals to community resources to decrease the possibility of re-admission.

Another compelling impetus for course development was to ensure that the curriculum conformed with Minnesota's Professional Nurse Practice Act (Minnesota Statute 148.211), which articulates the registered nurses's responsibility for "case finding and referral to other health resources." Newly implemented Minnesota Board of Nursing Program Approval Rules require that all students be evaluated for the following nursing abilities:

Section E   REFERRAL TO HEALTH RESOURCES
              "to identify available health resources which match a patient's needs and desires; and provide necessary information to patient and health resources."

Section K   HEALTH NEEDS OF FAMILIES
              " . . . to collect and interpret data pertaining to a family's structure and function in relation to health needs; and make a plan to assist a family to achieve a health goal."

Section L   HEALTH NEEDS OF COMMUNITIES WHICH AFFECT INDIVIDUAL'S HEALTH
              " . . . collect and interpret data pertaining to a community's population and environment in terms of the community's effects on an individual's health and make a plan for modifying a condition within the community which affects the health of an individual."

Prior to introducing the "Nurse in the Community" course, our curriculum did not include the required "family" or "community" emphases. Content on referrals was interspersed throughout the curriculum but concepts of discharge planning and continuity of care were not well-developed. Faculty believed that the program could be vulnerable in a Board of Nursing review process unless these concepts were strengthened and expanded.

Philosophically, the Inver Hills-Lakewood faculty had long believed that education must be proactive in implementing curriculum revisions that anticipate or parallel changes in the health care delivery system. They were convinced that ADN curricula must be revised to include concepts that would enable graduates to deal with the realities of an inpatient prospective payment health care system. Specifically, this meant expanding the graduates' learning outcomes to include knowledge of basic community health concepts, home care and community resources, and skills in discharge planning and referrals.

COURSE DEVELOPMENT

To address these multiple needs and concerns, a task force of nursing faculty members was convened to recommend curriculum revisions that would prepare graduates to function more effectively in the rapidly changing health care system. A second charge was to ensure that the curriculum conformed to the Minnesota Board of Nursing Program Approval Rules that articulate specific theoretical and practice concepts. Task force deliberations continued for two academic quarters; eventually, the group recommended the development of a new course. They drafted preliminary objectives with expected learning outcomes centered on knowledge of community resources and ability to apply key elements of comprehensive discharge planning. Even at this early stage, the faculty were convinced that "continuity of care" must be the major curriculum emphasis as a response to the expected shortened hospital stay and greater level of acuity among discharged patients.

As the "Nurse and the Community" course was developed, conscientious attention was given to planning and implementing content and course requirements which were anchored in the program's conceptual framework. The knowledge base and skills included also had to be consistent with the "MANEC Statement of Nursing Competencies" developed in 1978 to describe our graduates' competencies (Metro Area Nursing Education Consortium Statement of Graduate Competencies, 1980).

Once the decision had been made to organize the content into a new and distinct community health course, one faculty member was assigned the task of specific course development. Her responsibilities included a review of the literature, delineation and validation of course objectives, recommendations of course requirements, and formatting and drafting a plan for course evaluation. The instructor and the program director also defended the proposed curriculum revision throughout the usual college Curriculum Committee review and approval process.

REVIEW OF THE LITERATURE

A review of the literature was undertaken in June 1983, to identify the extent to which basic community health concepts were being included in Associate Degree Nursing curricula. Findings revealed that much of the literature, at that time, was devoted to defining the current practice of Associate Degree nurses. It reflected the struggle of baccalaureate, Associate Degree, and practical nurse educators to define and defend their products. Several nation-wide "competency" identification efforts were reported, describing the knowledge and skills required by different levels of practitioners (NLN, 1978). The literature consistently reflected the view that community health concepts were appropriate only to the baccalaureate level of nursing education. No documentation could be found that other ADN programs were organizing these concepts into a separate course.

The literature review of current and projected trends in health care delivery was significant in that it helped to clarify some implications for preparing future health care providers. In the early 1980s, the most obvious concern related to health care was cost containment. Hospital care expenditures had increased at an alarming rate and government, business, and third-party payors sought various methods of maintaining or reducing costs. By 1983, most proposed methods involved prospective reimbursement plans (Curtin, 1983). The Tax Equity and Fiscal Responsibility Act of 1982, Public Law 97-248, mandated ongoing legislation that was expected to reduce Medicare and Medicaid payments by more than $14 billion between 1983 and 1985. This act triggered major changes in the financial management of provider agencies as well as in the delivery of alternative health services (Grimaldi, 1983).

The concept of "continuity of care" was conspicuously absent from the literature describing efforts of nurse educators to revise curricula in the early 1980s. Nursing faculties could not, at that time, realistically predict the impact that these legislative changes would have on nursing care. Health care economists, however, were projecting that quality discharge planning would become increasingly more crucial as patient care shifted from acute care setting to the home and community in an attempt to reduce costs (Williams, 1983). Several books focusing on continuity of care were identified, and S.R. Beatty's *Continuity of Care: The Hospital and the Community* was particularly helpful in the initial formulation of course objectives.

COURSE OBJECTIVES

Reviewing the literature on current health care trends and relating these trends to nursing practice was an important step in identifying the foci of course content. The following five objectives were developed as a tentative framework for course content:

1. Gain knowledge of basic community health concepts.
2. Identify individual and family situations that require referral to community agencies.
3. Become aware of services that are appropriate and available for referral in the community.
4. Utilize steps in the referral process.
5. Given a discharge plan, identify community resources for referral.

In order to validate these objectives, structured interviews were conducted with nurses employed in a variety of work settings in June and July 1983. From each objective, a question or questions were devised to explore the opinions of employed nurses, identifying the knowledge and skills pertinent for the Associate Degree graduate caring for hospitalized patients. Those interviewed were not a random sample but included 12 nurses from two states working as public health nurses, staff nurses, discharge planners, administrators, and educators.

Several common themes and concerns were voiced by most of these individuals. All expressed concern related to the increased need for comprehensive discharge planning due to shorter hospital stay. Most of those interviewed believed that hospital nurses did not have adequate knowledge of appropriate, available community resources for referral. Both public health and hospital staff nurses described frustration in working within a system suffering from lack of continuity of care between hospital and community. Many cited a major area of difficulty as lack of information regarding available community services and poor communication between provider and facilities. The feedback from the interviews further substantiated the need to focus the course on continuity of care between hospital and community.

Final course objectives were revised based on conclusions drawn from the literature, interviews with nurses in the validation process, and Board of Nursing requirements. They are:

1. Define community, culture, family, case finding, health counseling, health promotion, health protection, prevention, referral process, and discharge planning.
2. Describe roles of the nurse as related to the community.
3. Identify cultural characteristics of four ethnic groups within our community and implications for nursing care.
4. Describe components of family assessment and identify components in a hypothetical family situation.
5. Describe components of community assessment and identify demographic information of the community.
6. Apply knowledge of the infectious cycle to individual and community health, using AIDS as a clinical case study.
7. Identify common community resources available to individuals throughout the life cycle.
8. Identify common community resources available for individuals with long-term or chronic illness.
9. Identify common community resources available for families or individuals in crisis.
10. Identify steps of a referral process and write a referral for a hospitalized patient.
11. Given a discharge plan, identify appropriate community resources for referral.
12. Identify current issues (state or national) where legislation impacts on nursing.

COURSE REQUIREMENTS

There are three components to the course: a didactic portion presenting theory, an observational clinical experience, and a segment focusing on discharge planning and the referral process. Theoretical content is presented by lecturers and guest speakers from the community, with objectives determining specific content areas. The overall intent of the theory portion is to provide the future technical nurse with information about how the health of the hospitalized individual is maximized by increasing continuity of care between health care providers.

Using established guidelines and specific objectives, students arrange their own observational clinical experience at any community agency or service that might be utilized in discharge planning or referrals. Observational experiences must have prior approval of the instructor and a paper is required to describe how the objectives are met. The visit may include an interview of agency employee/s (preferably a nurse) or observation of the direct services provided by the agency. Students typically choose to visit support groups, outpatient clinics, health education services, and home health care agencies. The site chosen dictates much variability in the experience of individual students, but the primary goal of this experience, to expose the student to the diversity of community resources available, is achieved.

Discharge planning comprises the third component of the course. Students are required to complete a discharge plan and referral for one of the patients they care for during the hospital clinical rotation portion of the nursing core course. In addition, the student develops a nursing care plan focusing on the needs of the patient at discharge.

EVALUATION

Evaluation has been an integral and dynamic aspect of the "Nurse and the Community" course. Since 1984, over 1,000 enrollees have completed the standard course evaluation form. Students have consistently rated the content on family assessment, infectious cycle and AIDS, transcultural nursing, and legislative issues as most applicable to clinical practice. Students identified original content on the infectious cycle as repetitive resulting in a revised course objective applying knowledge of communicable disease, using an AIDS case study. The students also requested additional specific information on the prospective payment system, diagnosis related groups, and continuing impact health care delivery systems have on the practice of technical nursing. Lecture content was revised accordingly.

Faculty have participated in course revision, particularly in the discharge planning segment. Students and community agencies also responded with suggestions to revise the discharge planning segment. As a result, the focus of this content was changed from a theoretical construct to a clinical application assignment. Nurse clinicians and community health practitioners have been generous and supportive in providing continual feedback and in mentoring at sites for the observational experiences. In the clinical setting, faculty observe that students are recognizing the importance of continuity of care and that discharge planning begins with patient admission. Course evaluation has been an ongoing process, incorporating student, faculty, and community input in an attempt to update course content and theory.

CONCLUSION

In the past eight years, the health care system and nursing practice have been greatly impacted by the federally mandated prospective payment system. Nursing education has a responsibility to implement curriculum changes that will address the realities of early discharge but will maintain and improve the quality of care provided by its graduates. Associate Degree nurses with increased knowledge of community health concepts and services and skills in discharge planning and implementing appropriate referrals will practice more competently, maintaining continuity of care among acute, community, and home settings.

REFERENCES

Competency of the AD nurse on entry into practice. (1978). NLN Division of AD Programs. Publication # 231731.

Curtin, L. (1983). Determining cost of nursing services per DRG. *Nursing Management, 14*(4), 16–20.

Grimaldi, P. (1983). Public Law 97-248:The implication of prospective payment schedules. *Nursing Management, 14*(2), 25–27.

MANEC Statement of Nursing Competencies. (1980, April). Metro Area Nursing Education Consortium funded by United States Department of Health, Education and Welfare.

Williams, M. (1983). DRG's—A primer. *Nursing Economics, 1,* 135–137.

11

Educational Accountability for an Aging Society

Vivian E. Ott*

*I*n 1985, the American Association of Retired Persons (AARP) published a report describing the extraordinary increase in the number of Americans age 65 and older. In 1960, this segment of the U.S. population numbered 16.78 million or 9.2 percent of the entire population. By 1984, the percentage was 11.9 and the AARP predicts that in the year 2030, 20–22 percent of the entire U.S. population will be age 65 and older (Connors, 1989).

The current societal trend toward aging and implications for health care delivery emphasize the need for gerontological nursing curriculum. Many professional nursing organizations such as the American Nurses Association (ANA) and the National League for Nursing (NLN) issued directives to all nursing programs urging implementation of gerontological curriculum. In response to these directives, many nursing programs developed gerontological curriculum to remain accountable to societal needs, especially those of an aging society.

---

* I thank my colleague and co-evaluator Myrian Works for her dedication to the evaluation project and valuable advice in preparing this manuscript.

This chapter addresses the rationale for remaining educationally accountable, identifies an evaluation paradigm with which to assess a program's accountability, and shares what I consider the embryonic phase of gerontological curriculum development at my institution, Roane State Community College.

DISCUSSION

Definition and Examples of Accountability

The *Random House College Dictionary* (1984) defines the term *accountable* as: (a)"subject to the obligation to report, explain, or justify something; responsible, answerable; and (b) capable of being explained; explicable" (p. 10). Synonyms for the term include *liable, blameworthy, answerable, responsible,* and *chargeable* (Random House Thesaurus, 1984, p. 19). The term *answerable* conveys my position that we as nursing educators possess answers to the needs of an aging society.

To whom and for what are we accountable? Historically or in retrospect, one of the earliest reasons for "creating" education was to facilitate the passage of "cultural heritage from one generation to the next" (Hartoonian, 1991, p. 23). Growing out of such a context, education became inundated with the expressions of social norms and values. Having been created, so to speak, by the people for the express use of the people, education and its educators became accountable to society.

Bahr (1988) credited Florence Nightingale with creating a profession uniquely responsive to societal mandates; consequently, health care, which is considered a right for everyone, is accountable to the general public. Accountability implies health care professionals are adequately trained to deal with all societal health care needs.

Introspectively, I envision nursing educators as accountable to: themselves in the execution of daily activities according to personal philosophies of nursing; students in preparing them to render capable and willing service; institutions (both academic and practice) in maintaining cost-effectiveness while not sacrificing quality and in maximizing their customer responsiveness; their profession in balancing the expectations of both educators and practitioners and in the execution of our "moral duty to safeguard a patient's rights" (Freel,

1990, p. 571); and to society (individuals and collective whole) in pursuit of adequate, specialized care for those with a variety of needs, in a variety of settings.

Tanner (1992), in an editorial for the *Journal of Nursing Education,* addressed the prospective need for educational accountability. She advocated assisting students to analyze societal issues and to become active citizens and spokespersons for a variety of health-related social issues. She concluded her editorial by challenging educators to help students adopt professional roles as agents and leaders advocating social change.

Rationale

Why become educationally accountable to society for issues raised by an aging population? Although I will not debate the rationale so eloquently proffered by my colleagues for the inclusion of gerontological curriculum into nursing education (Atchison & Bryant, 1988; Bahr, 1987; Edel, 1986), I will delineate three rationales as noted in nursing literature.

The first rationale for becoming educationally accountable reflects what Tom Peters (1987) described as customer responsiveness. As a business specialist, Peters predicted that, "Success in health-care will go to those who add value by developing customized products or services that create new market niches" (p. 48). As nursing educators, we need to join with our practitioner colleagues in determining the breadth, length, and height of our responsibility and accountability toward our customers and in establishing for ourselves a niche in the marketplace.

The second rationale reveals the need for specific knowledge concerning the aging patient as nurses assess, plan, implement, and evaluate the delivery of care and services to this population.

The third rationale addresses nursing's need to remain abreast with activities engaged in by other disciplines and to "protect" nursing, so to speak, from those graduating with degrees in sociology, social work, ethics, and family studies, which also prepared them to meet the needs of an aging society. Inclusive here is another reason for becoming proactive: to stem society's current impatience with the educational system. Such impatience grows whenever society perceives educators as not adequately addressing important issues, although several examples do exist that exemplify society's ability to enact rules and laws by which accountability is exacted and extracted from the educational system. Responding to such mandates provides opportunity for knee-jerk reactive rather than proactive endeavors by the profession.

Evaluation Paradigm

Having established the need for being educationally accountable to society, how can nursing faculties determine whether their curricula adequately address the needs of a more and more aging society? Becoming involved in evaluating the curriculum provides powerful indicators of the degree to which the curriculum responds to the perceived needs of the customers or society at large. To allow curriculum development and evaluation to occur simultaneously, however, is somewhat more complex and requires an appropriate, if initial evaluation framework. Thus, we turned to Bellon and Handler's (1982) Status Study. A Status Study assists educators in describing the current status of a particular program or curriculum and ends with recommendations to aid in the development of improvement plans. Bellon and Handler recommended that such a study describe the goals, organization, operations, and outcomes of a particular program in question.

A Status Study is an eclectic evaluation framework drawn from aspects of goal-driven frameworks as proposed by Tyler, Provus, and Hammond, and management with its program, planning, budgeting systems (PPBS); goal-free framework by Scriven; decision management framework by Stufflebeam—content, input, process, and products (CIPP); professional judgment frameworks by Stake, Rippey, and Eisner; and the adversary framework by Wolf (Barrow, 1984; Guba & Lincoln, 1981; Orlosky & Smith, 1978).

When analyzing the *goals* and philosophy statements of a particular program, evaluative activities center on information-gathering efforts such as interviewing persons involved in the program and content analysis. It is also important to determine the emphasis placed on goals and the belief in and value attached to a particular goal or set of goals.

While evaluating the *organization,* educators must systematically examine the current functioning of the entire organization, including funding sources, roles and responsibilities of individual players, communication patterns, and program offerings by other departments. Evaluation concerns whether the program or curriculum in question has an apparent relationship to overall goals and priorities established by the parent organization.

To accurately evaluate the curriculum, the Status Study requires descriptions of day-to-day activities or the *operations*. This allows educators to assess how well current philosophy, goals, and priorities translate into action on a daily basis. Goals and priorities should be evident in written descriptions of classroom events and student assignments. The actual class time devoted to a particular segment of the curriculum strongly indicates the faculty's commitment to the established goal(s). Also included in the description of a curriculum's operation is the examination of staff development.

The last segment of a Status Study investigates the *outcomes* of the curriculum. How well do students score on evaluation tools regarding the curriculum? What tools exist that measure the outcome of particular goals set? Educators also examine the possible side effects of a curriculum; for example, changes in students' attitudes or career interests.

RESULTS

The following highlights our Status Study findings and resulting recommendations for curriculum improvement. Keep in mind that these recommendations and the ensuing project stem from our evaluation findings and may not be applicable to another setting (Table 1). Evaluation results, unlike research, are not generalizable; therefore, I do not advocate that Associate Degree nursing programs assimilate our

---

Table 1
Curriculum Revision Recommendations

Future gerontological curriculum revisions should:

1. Include gerontological curriculum throughout the 2-year program.
2. Expose students to the "well" older adult and related concepts before presenting issues relating to the chronically "ill" older adult.
3. Incorporate experiential learning methods into the curriculum.
4. Provide theoretical learning via self-paced independent study packets.
5. Arrange a six-week clinical rotation for first-year students and a four-week rotation for second-year students.

---

project without first engaging in similar evaluation efforts. Our Status Study allowed us to look at the goals currently in place for gerontological curriculum, observe the transactions occurring on a day-to-day basis, and analyze the curriculum outcomes.

Goals

We began our evaluation by analyzing curricular content and the emphasis placed on goal statements. We assumed our program addressed gerontological issues because one of the curricular threads—"Life Cycle"—is described by an outcome objective stating: "The student will apply principles of growth and development in providing nursing care to individuals and families in various stages of the life cycle" (RSCC, 1991, p. 64). Furthermore, each semester's course description states that theory and application of nursing skills will address the needs of "individuals at various stages throughout the life cycle."

As we explored the emphasis placed during fundamental, medical-surgical, and psychiatric lectures on the curricular thread—"Life Cycle"—we noted that very few content objectives (e.g., one out of 78 med-surg objectives) related to the older adult and the aging process. Quiz questions, eliciting student knowledge regarding gerontological content, ranged from 4 to 11 percent of any given quiz. Of the textbooks used, only 142 pages or 5.8 percent of the 2,439 pages required for class preparation pertained to the care of older adults. These results amplify the marginal inclusion of gerontological components in our curriculum.

Organization

Reviewing the organizational support for gerontological emphasis revealed no specific class offering, either for credit or non-credit, dealing with the issues of aging. Three courses, offered by the psychology, sociology, and humanities departments, according to their descriptions, dealt with aging or gerontological issues peripherally, that is, as a subcomponent. The audio-visual department and library had 15 tapes, 36 books, and 2 journals, *Geriatric Nursing* and *Modern Maturity*, that addressed geriatric issues. While resources may be lacking, we do have the support of our program director in establishing stronger gerontological emphasis within our curriculum.

Bellon and Handler (1982) recommended evaluating the organization's financial support of a particular program; for example, nursing programs at our institution receiving substantial funding are academic development, the writing center, and the most recently developed program—technological improvement. Assessing the organization's patterns of resource allocation is especially helpful in depicting the priority status held by the program being evaluated. If organizational support is lacking, nursing educators may recommend a strategic plan outlining how to strengthen existing support or they may opt not to proceed with curriculum development and improvement until better support is obtained.

Operations

Although we chose not to conduct in-classroom observations for evidence of gerontological content inclusion, we did tally the ages of patients assigned to students during their medical-surgical hospital rotations. Of the four rotations sampled, the average patient age was 64.8 years. During the students' extended care rotation (home health visitation), they read "A Fresh Look at Assessing the Elderly," by Andresen (1989), and wrote papers addressing the issues of aging. A future evaluative activity will elicit the students' perceptions regarding lecture coverage of gerontological content.

Another area descriptive of a curriculum's operation is the examination of staff development. In this regard, my colleague and I attended the Southern Regional Education Board workshop, held in Atlanta, in 1991, "Faculty Preparation for Teaching Gerontological Nursing." Due to statewide cutbacks on staff development funding, we financed this trip ourselves. However, our institution did agree to fund my colleague's tuition when she enrolled in a gerontological issues class at the University of Tennessee.

Outcomes

Our initial evaluation of outcomes included administering Palmore's (1977) "Facts on Aging, A Short Quiz" both to first-year and second-year students and tallying employment trends of graduates. The Palmore Quiz is a 25-item true-or-false quiz that assesses knowledge regarding physical, mental, and social facts along with misconceptions

Table 2
Palmore's "Facts on Aging" Quiz: Differentiating Results
According to Students' Desire to Work in Geriatrics

First Year		Second Year	
Yes	*No*	*Yes*	*No*
N: 15 (26%)	42	17 (40%)	25
M: 65.5%	50%	62.7%	58.9%
R: 33–100%	33–91.7%	41.7–91.7%	33.83%

regarding the elderly. Fifty-seven first-year students responded to our survey and attained a sample quiz average of 57.8 percent. Forty-two second-year students participated and attained a sample average of 61 percent.

Quiz results placed our students as scoring lower than participants in studies conducted by Greenhill and Baker (1986), Harrison and Novak (1988), and Kline and Kline (1991), all of whom used Palmore's Aging Quiz to determine participants' baseline knowledge. We further differentiated quiz results according to the students' stated desire for working with older adults (see Table 2).

Our tally of graduates' initial place of employment indicated that, out of 205 graduates (1987–1991), six (2.9%) went into extended-care facilities (nursing homes), and 14 (6.8%) went into home health; yet only a negligible curricular emphasis is on gerontology and home health issues. However, while one-third of medical-surgical curriculum is devoted to pediatric concepts, only seven graduates (3.4%) selected this field. This dichotomy in curriculum selection does not reflect the current and future needs of our "customers."

Needs Assessment

With the knowledge gained from content analysis supporting some of our recommendations, my colleague and I conducted a needs assessment to determine further what curricular emphasis our customers/constituents desired. Our survey, divided into four short sections, asked for input regarding: (1) theoretical content, (2) curricular emphasis of content, (3) criteria for clinical experiences, and (4) clinical skills. We disseminated this survey to all directors of nursing (DONs) represented on our Advisory Council and to the DONs of various health care facilities (e.g., nursing homes, extended care, home health).

According to our survey (which had a 75% return rate), the *most* important theoretical content areas for curricular inclusion were: (1) health assessment of older adults and (2) the older adult's normal growth and development. Areas of *least* importance to our constituents were: (1) cultural variations affecting health care of older adults and (2) demographics of older adults. Most of the respondents (80%) felt it was "very important" or "important" for students to be exposed to the well older adult prior to the chronically ill.

According to our survey, curricular emphasis to be placed on various theoretical components should center on: (1) common health problems and their treatment, and dealing with chronic illness; (2) role and function of the nurse in gerontology; and (3) normal growth and development. The curricular areas needing the *least* amount of curricular emphasis were: (1) demographics of older adults and political issues affecting older adults and (2) cultural variations affecting health care.

Survey responses indicating the importance of various clinical experience criteria showed that: (1) direct contact with older adults, (2) access to a diverse older adult population, (3) diversity of tasks and experiences, and (4) expert supervision were, in the order presented, the most important. The clinical criteria "utilization of a variety of agencies and organizations" was deemed least important. When asked which clinical skills were important in working with the older adult, all 24 responders indicated that the two *most* important skills would be the assessment and identification of normal versus abnormal changes in aging.

Although our needs assessment results may differ from those published by Kuehn (1991), Tollett and Thornby (1982), Verderber and Kick (1990), and many others, we maintain that because of our evaluative efforts, our curriculum suits the needs of all constituents—employers, students, and the elderly.

Curriculum Design

Based on our Status Study findings and needs assessment results, the recommendations listed in Table 2 assisted us with curriculum planning. The ensuing nursing curriculum revisions expose students to the concepts of wellness and older adults within a six-week clinical rotation the first year and the concepts of chronic illness in a four-week rotation the second year. The six- and four-week time frames are based on the length of the other rotations during those semesters.

Corresponding with each clinical component, students engage in completing an independent study packet containing theoretical concepts. We currently incorporate independent study packets into a cardiac and an extended care rotation. Successful use of independent learning in the areas mentioned lead us to believe that additional independent packets would continue to meet the needs of our student population.

First-year clinical gerontological rotation allows students, in retirement facilities, community centers, or nursing home settings, to observe and identify a client's needs for wellness promotion. During their sessions, students implement a wellness teaching plan. Concurrent with clinical observations, students complete theoretical components such as physiology of aging, societal attitudes, sensory changes, and normal nutritional needs.

During the eight days spent in the nursing home working with older adults and their chronic illnesses, second-year students conduct head-to-toe physical examinations, medication interaction assessments, one interdisciplinary conference, and a nutritional assessment and evaluation, and they implement rehabilitation principles. Independent study theoretical components include common health problems and their treatment, ethical issues, and role and function of the gerontological nurse. The independent study packets contain an eclectic assortment of journal and textbook readings, audio-visual assignments, and experiential learning.

CONCLUSION

My colleague and I believe an Associate Degree nursing curriculum effectively provides students with marketable skills and the ability to work as functional members of society. To this end, educational accountability has been maintained. However, substantial evidence exists indicating current curricular emphasis may not be sufficient when addressing the future needs of an aging society and of nursing graduates. We maintain that engaging in a Status Study and needs assessment allowed our faculty to formulate a gerontological curriculum that addresses our accountability to an aging society, our constituents, our graduates, and our profession. We hope that future graduates will be capable and willing to address the issues of an aging society. We at Roane State want to be part of what Ebersole (1990) described as the "political and social reform that will better serve the aged in our health-care system" (p. 61).

REFERENCES

Andresen, G.P. (1989, June). A fresh look at assessing the elderly. *RN, 28–40.*

Atchison, J., & Bryant, B. (1988). Ageism in the nursing curricula. *Journal of Nursing Science and Practice, 1*(1), 1–2.

Bahr, R.T. (1987). Adding to the educational agenda. *Journal of Gerontological Nursing, 13*(3), 6–11.

Bahr, R.T. (1988). Ethical issues within the gerontological nursing curriculum. Nursing Special Project Grant (D 10 NU 24299-01). Atlanta, GA: Southern Regional Education Board.

Barrow, R. (1984). Curriculum evaluation. In *Giving teaching back to teachers* (pp. 230–250). Sussex, NJ: Wheatsheaf Books, LTD.

Bellon, J.J., & Handler, J.R. (1982). *Curriculum development and evaluation. A design for improvement.* Dubuque, IA: Kendall/Hunt.

Connors, H.R. (1989). Impact evaluation of a statewide continuing education program. *The Journal of Continuing Education in Nursing, 20*(2), 64–69.

Ebersole, P. (1990). The future of gerontic nursing. *Imprint, 37*(4), 59–61.

Edel, M. (1986). Recognize gerontological content. *Journal of Gerontological Nursing, 12*(10), 28–32.

Flexner, S.B., & Stein, J. (Eds.). (1984). *The Random House college dictionary* (Revised Edition). New York: Random House.

Freel, M. (1990). Truth telling. In J.C. McCloskey & H.K. Grace (Eds.), *Current Issues in Nursing* (p. 571). St. Louis: C.V. Mosby.

Greenhill, D., & Baker, M. (1986). The effects of a well older adult clinical experience on students' knowledge and attitudes. *Journal of Nursing Education, 25*(4), 145–147.

Guba, E.G., & Lincoln, Y.S. (1981). A new approach to evaluation. In *Effective evaluation.* Washington DC: Jossey-Bass.

Harrison, L., & Novak, D. (1988). Evaluation of a gerontological nursing continuing education programme: Effect on nurses' knowledge and attitudes and on patients' perceptions and satisfaction. *Journal of Advanced Nursing, 13*(5), 684–692.

Hartoonian, M. (1991). Good education is bad politics: Practices and principles of school reform. *Social Education, 55*(1), 22–23, 65.

Kline, T., & Kline, D. (1991). Identification of response bias on two knowledge of aging questionnaires by use of randomized tests. *Gerontology & Geriatrics Education, 11*(4), 67–75.

Kuehn, A. (1991). Essential gerontological content for the associate degree nursing curriculum: A national study. *Journal of Gerontological Nursing, 17*(8), 20–27.

Orlosky, D.E., & Smith, B.O. (1978). Methods of curriculum evaluation. In *Curriculum Development: Issues and Insights* (pp. 392–417). Chicago: Rand McNally College Publishing Company.

Palmore, E. (1977). Facts on aging: A short quiz. *The Gerontologist, 17*(4), 315–320.

Peters, T. (1987). Creating total customer responsiveness. *Thriving on chaos.* New York: Knopf.

Roane State Community College (RSCC) (1991). *Self-study for NLN Reaccreditation.* Harriman, TN: Nursing Department Faculty.

Stein, J., & Flexner, S.B. (Eds). (1984). *The Random House thesaurus* (college edition). New York: Random House.

Tanner, C.A. (1992). Education as a social responsibility. *Journal of Nursing Education, 31*(1), 3.

Tollett, S., & Thornby, J. (1982). Geriatric and gerontology nursing curricular threads. *Journal of Nursing Education, 21*(6), 16–23.

Verderber, D., & Kick, E. (1990). Gerontological curriculum in schools of nursing. *Journal of Nursing Education, 29*(8), 355–361.

12

The Prospective of Long-Term Care Educational Partnerships: An Essential Community Collaboration

Mary Ann Anderson
Gail Cobe

*T*his occasion of the 40th anniversary of Associate Degree Nursing education is significant. I appreciate the fact that the Community College-Nursing Home Partnership Project is part of this celebration. It is appropriate because this project has contributed to the recent history of Associate Degree nursing.

We are presenting this chapter as two of the original six coordinators for the W. K. Kellogg funded Community College-Nursing Home Partnership, "Improving Care Through Education Project." This project was funded for six associate schools nationally: Ohlone College, Fremont, California; Shoreline Community College, Seattle, Washington; Weber State University, Ogden, Utah; Triton College, Riverside, Illinois; Community College of Philadelphia, Philadelphia, Pennsylvania; and Valencia Community College, Orlando, Florida.

The origin of the project was to define methodologies for nursing education to utilize in addressing the geriatric imperative in this nation within the framework of the curriculum revolution in nursing. In other words, how to educate student nurses to give effective care to frail elderly clients without adding hours to curricula that are already overloaded. In this sixth year of the project, each of the six original schools involved remain active participants. In addition, they have grown by developing a cadre of other member schools who participate in the project with their support and mentoring.

EDUCATING FOR THE YEAR 2000

The impetus for the Community College-Nursing Home Partnership Project is based on the fact that the student nurse of the year 2000 will be required by society to be skilled in giving care to elder clients on a level of sophistication that has not existed in nursing prior to this decade. The actual practice of nursing will drive education in the future as it has in the past, making educational partnerships essential to effective curricular content.

In a focused effort to address this current yet prospective need, the Community College-Nursing Home Partnership Project funded by the W. K. Kellogg Foundation has developed methodologies and strategies for educational partnerships with long-term care facilities. The results of such partnerships in the six Associate Degree Nursing (ADN) project schools have been diverse and positive. The diversity allows for application of the process to a wide variety of educational settings.

FACULTY ADVANTAGES

The advantages to ADN faculty are numerous. First, the curriculum is pertinent to the needs of the profession. The project schools have made curriculum pertinent without adding hours to curricula that are already heavy. The key here has been utilization of the long-term care facility as a well-designed clinical experience. Also important is the placement of faculty and students in the nursing facility, which is focused on concepts defined by the project as "best taught" in long-term care, including "best-taught" skills critical to RN functioning in every clinical setting.

The educational partnerships that are developed provide faculty with resources in gerontological nursing that otherwise have not been available. We must remember that clinical experts in nursing homes are a resource; they are able and eager to provide theoretical and clinical experiences in support of the faculty needs.

An essential part of this chapter is the presentation of information that will facilitate your ability to teach elder care in the long-term care setting effectively. Yet, you might wonder, "Why do I need to teach that content?" The national statistics on the aging of America make it clear why gerontological nursing is being recognized as essential content for every nursing curriculum.

Another question might be, "Why does it have to be done in long-term care when over 50 percent of my patients in the hospital are over age 65?" The entire focus of the Community College-Nursing Home Partnership Project goes beyond just giving care to frail elders; it interfaces very closely with the personae of professional nursing and the definition of skills best taught in specific clinical settings. There is knowledge to impart and skills to be taught that are most effectively done in the nursing home environment. For many faculty this is new and sometimes difficult to accept.

PROFESSIONAL VALUING

An unplanned benefit of placing students and faculty in long-term care facilities directly relates to professional valuing. The Community College-Nursing Home Partnership has helped nursing faculty to learn to value their colleagues in the nursing home. This is a new experience for many nursing home professionals. In spite of the autonomy, lack of immediate medical intervention, and, oftentimes, lack of another licensed professional to assist with assessment and subsequent decision making, nursing home registered nurses have been considered by some in the profession as "less than adequate" professionals. When faculty members have gone to these experts with an educational partnership as the goal, very positive things have happened, most significantly *professional valuing.*

Faculty who work with the project have experienced the dedication of long-term care nurses, noted their strengths, and joined their struggle to provide care for the frail elderly. This mutual respect encourages both faculty and clinical nurses to find meaningful learning experiences that will serve students regardless of where they practice.

Allow me to relate a story to help you understand what type of learning can happen when students are placed in long-term care (LTC) facilities. At Weber State University, we have 140 freshmen on our main campus each fall. There are only two hospitals in the city and it is obvious that they cannot accommodate all of the freshmen for the course in fundamentals of nursing. As a result, we place fundamentals students in LTC facilities. This is a story about one of those students.

The clinical instructor for the course in fundamentals of nursing works in a focused way to teach her students the nursing process. As a result of that instruction, each student has to identify a need for his or her resident by the third day of clinical work and on day five he or she is to have the problem solved in such a way that he or she can meet the need for the resident. One student went directly to her resident and asked her, "What can I do for you that no one else can do?"

The resident burst into tears and after being calmed somewhat by the student said, "I want to see my dog. I have not seen him since I came to the nursing home."

The student was excited to have a project to work on and also noticed that it seemed somewhat easy. She went back to her instructor and told her of the plan. She had enough experience with dogs to recognize that she needed permission to bring the animal into the nursing facility and planned with the director of nursing the course of action she would take if the dog misbehaved because of his excitement.

Once approval was granted for all possible dog-related problems, the student called the resident's husband and told him of her plan. The husband explained that he could not bring the dog to the nursing home because he did not drive and the taxi company would only let seeing eye dogs into their vehicles. The student was not daunted by this obstacle and after being referred by her instructor to the social service worker, she made several calls to community service agencies. She not only brought the dog for a visit to her resident, but he had a clip and shampoo before he came! Oh, yes, the dog did "have an accident," not on the floor as anticipated, but right in his mistresses bed!

When this freshman student told me about her experience, she was very animated and proud of what she had accomplished. I asked her if she could feel the empowerment that had come from that experience. I was not surprised when she did not know the verbal definition of empowerment; it was exciting to explain it to her with her recent experience as an excellent example! Do you use the concept? This was a freshman student who learned about professional empowerment because of opportunities for learning that are available in the slower paced, more interdisciplinary, focused nursing facility.

DESIGNING A CURRICULUM

Nursing facilities are *not* second-class hospitals. Instead, they are unique health care settings where learning for students can take place in a proactive style rather than the traditional reactive style that is seen in the acute-care environment. In an effort to capitalize on the learning that can take place in this specialized setting, the Community College-Nursing Home Partnership Project decided to do a curriculum evaluation known by the acronym DACum, which means Designing A Curriculum. In this case, it was designing a curriculum based on what is needed to be taught to a future RN in order for that RN to be effective in the long-term care setting. Through the DACum process, the national project also was able to define the skills that are best taught in long-term care facilities.

In order to accomplish this task, 12 representative directors of nursing working in partnership nursing homes from across the nation gathered in Chicago in August of 1988. They completed a DACum during an intensive two days. The DACum process uses a modified brainstorming approach. After hours of discussion guided by a facilitator, these clinical nursing leaders identified and sequenced 300 skills/behaviors that were critical to the work done in nursing facilities. Several analyses by project faculty followed until four categories with 22 specific competencies "best taught" in a long-term setting emerged (see Table 1 for a complete list). The four main categories are:

1. Practice rehabilitation nursing skills.
2. Perform physical assessments.
3. Manage the living environment.
4. Exhibit management skills.

During examination of these competencies, the national project faculty were convinced that we owed students a clinical experience in a nursing home. It also was determined that this was appropriate as a well-designed, second-year experience. The complex residents in long-term care require the skills of a second-year student. In situations where freshmen use the nursing facility, the instructor has a strong challenge to not overwhelm the students with the complexity of institutionalized, frail, elderly clients.

Table 1
Competencies Best Taught in the Nursing Home

PERFORM ASSESSMENT OF RESIDENT

- Assess current mental status
- Assess functional (ADL and instrumental) abilities
- Differentiate normal aging process from disease process
- Recognize age-related differences in disease processes
- Value goals that maintain functional ability

PRACTICE REHABILITATION NURSING

- Define restorative goals
- Elicit active participation of resident in restorative program
- Facilitate choices to decrease learned helplessness
- Promote independence of ADLs
- Initiate bowel and bladder training
- Implement contracture prevention methods
- Evaluate effectiveness of restorative programs
- Implement group therapies, e.g., reality orientation, memory enhancement, reminiscing

MANAGE THE LIVING ENVIRONMENT

- Allow resident to continue previous lifestyle to degree possible
- Provide comfortable, homelike environment for socialization
- Plan room arrangement to facilitate resident needs
- Reduce environmental stress, e.g., noise, isolation, lighting, roommate
- Provide opportunities for expression of ethnic and cultural practices for residents
- Provide for sexual expression of residents
- Initiate intervention to deal with combative residents
- Assist families to cope with unrealistic expectations, guilt, anger

EXHIBIT MANAGEMENT SKILLS

- Adopt leadership style appropriate to situation
- Delegate appropriately
- Resolve problems utilizing problem-solving skills over an extended period of time
- Update care plan

PARTNERSHIPS

If nursing is to meet the current challenges and those of the next decade, it cannot chance to divide its energies. Strength comes from unity. As nurses, we must eliminate the mind set that pits service against education, baccalaureate education against Associate Degree education, student against faculty, and acute care against long-term care. The "we-they" syndrome and the "one-upmanship" game have no place in nursing.

Nursing is about doing nurses' work. It is about promoting health, maintaining function, and ensuring dignity for those in decline. The Community College-Nursing Home Partnership has learned a great deal about "nursing's work" and about gaining strength from unity. It has developed partnerships between nurse educators and nurse providers, between community colleges and nursing homes, and between faculty and students.

Project school faculty, after being immersed in the nursing home, became aware that there has been a lack of contact, communication, and collaboration that has inadvertently fostered negative images of the profession. When faculty and students exclude nursing staff in planning the provision of care for a select group of residents, the message is "collaboration is a sometime thing." Subtle messages that educators occasionally give to students diminish the profession. These seem to be based on society's negative mores regarding aging people and those who give them care. Nursing faculty have not sought out learning experiences in nursing facilities in the past and in this way or, perhaps, because of it, they have contributed to the devaluing of geriatric caregivers along with devaluing the elderly.

Although it seems inappropriate to compare nursing with medicine, when we do in this arena there are concepts to be learned. Rarely does a physician diminish his profession. Rarely in medicine does anyone hear the medical professor state that he or she cannot find role models for the medical student. Instead the medical professor demonstrates respect for colleagues in service regardless of specialty and setting.

THE ADVANTAGES

The nursing home is a rich environment for students and students enrich the home in return. Students teach nursing assistants and both they and residents benefit. Students learn to teach, communicate, facilitate teamwork, and delegate. Nursing assistants receive continuing education, participate at bedside rounds, are motivated, and have the opportunity to see "the making of a nurse."

Students and faculty alike begin to understand the "culture" of the nursing assistant and the "ethos" of the home. Nursing staff meet with faculty to discuss clinical issues and student learning experiences. In some project schools, staff have input into student evaluations. In all settings, the staff work toward helping the student meet the learning objectives.

Nursing homes and colleges have benefited from the partnership in many other ways: resources are shared; nursing home representatives sit on college advisory boards; books, videos, and professional periodicals are made available to all who are appropriate, and intergenerational programs have been developed. These latter programs involve partnerships among faculty of early childhood studies, preschoolers, and elders who reside in nursing homes. Partners meet on a regular basis for a planned activity and meal. During these times elders read, teach, and enjoy the children. Students and preschoolers learn about what it means to be old, and on occasion they learn about death. Bioethics Councils have been formed where nurse educators and care providers join together to manage the pressing ethical dilemmas faced when caring for elders.

As a result of the partnership, faculty teach differently. Individualizing care is a reality rather than an "ought to." The differences in priorities, pace, and focus of care in the nursing home, when compared to the acute setting, lead to a difference in assignments. Teaching the art of caring has grown in legitimacy. Faculty assume less of an evaluator/expert role and more of a mentor/colleague role. Without the acuity seen in the hospital, faculty are less stressed and autocratic, and students are less submissive. Both become more creative partners in the endeavors of education and nursing.

WHAT DOES IT LOOK LIKE?

In support of the adage, a picture is worth a thousand words, the National League for Nursing produced a video *Time to Care,* directed by Verle Waters, MS, RN, showing what a well-designed sophomore clinical experience in a nursing facility under the guidance of educational partners can look like. By watching this video; you will see firsthand the character and effect of the clinical experience on students, teachers, and other clients. You will like what you see.

A FINAL THOUGHT

The video, *Time to Care,* showed the learning that as faculty we hope to see in every student. It incorporated both the art and science of nursing based on the nursing process. As the last student in the video said, "It is a good idea for us to work in the nursing home. . . . " I agree with her. It is a good idea for students to work in the nursing home with faculty who are prepared to work in that setting as a partner to the professionals in the facility. Yet I have also talked about this topic long enough to recognize that some nursing professionals still believe that it is not necessary to place students in nursing facilities no matter how "well-designed" the experiences are! For those of you who feel this way, I have a final story to relate. A student who graduated from the Community College of Philadelphia went to work in an NICU in a large hospital in New York City. One year after graduation, she was sent the usual program evaluation form. This story is what she shared at that time.

This student indicated that she was working in NICU and commented that the skills she learned in how to communicate and work with the elderly was one of the most valuable aspects of her sophomore year. This may seem confusing without, however, the entire story. The patients for this new graduate were crack babies. The hospital had an organized grandparent program for the crack baby unit. This was a situation where volunteer elderly people would come to the unit and assist nurses by holding, rocking, and, in general, loving these crying and demanding babies. The new graduate commented on how most of the RNs were uncomfortable allowing the volunteer grandparents to hold and love the babies and, therefore, did not utilize them to the comfort of their patients. However, for this former student, there was no problem because she knew how to talk to and work with the elderly. She had learned to respect and value this age group while in school and naturally and eagerly incorporated them into her clinical practice.

A second thought she expressed was just as significant. Think for a moment to whom this nurse would discharge her little patients. It generally was not to the parents who were addicted to drugs. Most often it was to the grandparents.

This RN was able to practice successfully and on a higher level than some of her colleagues because she knew how to work with elderly people! I will say one more time: the skills taught while doing clinical learning in nursing facilities are skills that serve a registered nurse wherever he or she may work.

REFERENCES

Hammer, Rita M., & Tufts, Margaret A. (1985, September). Nursing's self image—Nursing education's responsibility. *Journal of Nursing Education, 24*(7), 280–283.

Tagliareni, E., Sherman, S., Waters, V., & Mengel, A. (1991, May). Participatory clinical education: Reconceptualizing the clinical learning environment. *Nursing & Health Care, 12*(5).

Walker, D. (1986, April). Nursing education and service: The payoffs of partnerships. *Nursing & Health Education,* 189–191.

13

Developing Management Skills Through a Preceptor-Based Experience in Community Nursing Homes

Patricia M. Bentz
Janice R. Ellis

*I*n 1988, as part of a curriculum revision that included goals of enhancing the teaching of gerontology, expanding upon the use of the nursing home as a clinical site, and teaching management concepts for nursing, the faculty at Shoreline Community College, Seattle, Washington, developed a preceptor-based management experience. The general goals were based on the faculty's recognition of the changing demographics of the population, the increasing need for nurses prepared to function in long-term care, and the imperative expressed by our colleagues who practice in nursing homes that all nurses must have management skills.

WHY CHOOSE A PRECEPTOR MODEL?

We chose to use a preceptor model for two major reasons. The first was the need for expert role models for students. We recognized that although faculty are experts in some areas, it is increasingly difficult for faculty to be experts everywhere they must teach. With a focus in a particular area, the staff nurse is an expert with regard to the particular patient population and with regard to the facility and the way in which it functions. Second, we wanted to provide students with individualized supervision. We believed that if we wanted students to operate in a management role, they would need immediate access to advice and supervision to maintain quality of care as well as quality in the work environment for others on the nursing team. With clinical groups of 10 students, it would be impossible for a faculty member to be this accessible.

In addition to these two major concerns, the faculty identified other reasons for constructing this experience. We wanted the experience to be located in a nursing home setting because we believed that management experiences were more available to students there. Also, we were committed to supporting the role of the nurse in long-term care. We believed that working in this role as a student would enhance respect for the role of the long-term care nurse and perhaps make a difference in career paths chosen by students. In our geographic area, we have many high-quality nursing homes, but none was large enough to have an entire clinical section work in management roles at one time. This meant that we could not have an instructor on-site at all times. We knew we would have to have students in several different facilities at the same time in order to provide that experience. Preceptors also provided an answer to this problem.

ROLES OF THE PARTICIPANTS

The principal participants in the Shoreline model included the nursing instructor, the staff nurse preceptor (SNP), and the nursing student. Since the preceptor-based experience was new to all involved, it was clear that a careful delineation of roles was necessary (Limon, Bargagliotti, & Spencer, 1982).

Initially, the nursing instructor serves as a coordinator—providing the director of nursing or staff development coordinator at the nursing home with the clinical schedule, the name(s) of the student(s) to be sent to the setting, and any other pertinent information. Lead time is important and should be established at the outset. In our case, the nursing homes indicated a need to have this information at least two months in advance to facilitate their scheduling.

During the actual clinical experience, the instructor adopts a "circuit rider" mode—traveling among the various nursing homes, serving as an observer, a mentor, and a problem solver. Faculty members who are working with a preceptor-based model must alter the way they have traditionally worked with students. Instructors provide support and guidance for preceptors and encourage students to relate to the preceptor for specific needs. Instructors need to step back and let the preceptor/student role be primary. One of the losses that faculty feel is in the role of expert with regard to the client. The SNP is clearly the expert in this situation and instructor must defer to that expertise. The instructor provides support to the SNP and the SNP-student relationship while the student is encouraged to collaborate with the SNP instead of the instructor (Hsieh & Knowles, 1990).

During on-campus clinical conferences, students are encouraged to discuss their experiences. In conferences, students learn from the experiences of students in other facilities. The faculty member continually encourages the students to solve their own problems and work out difficulties that arise without the intervention of the instructor.

The instructor may have the opportunity to participate in direct observation of the student, but that is not essential. The SNP serves as the primary person involved in direct observation of the student's activities. He or she identifies and provides opportunities for the student to perform specific skills and is encouraged to send the student to other departments or wings of the institution to accomplish this. In addition, the SNP provides ongoing oral and written feedback to the student, consulting with the instructor as needed. Preceptors are teachers, mentors, and evaluators for students.

The student is expected to identify his or her own learning needs, communicate them to the SNP, and plan with the SNP to meet those needs. The student works under the direct supervision of the SNP, with a view toward a collegial relationship—a relationship in which the instructor plays a minor role. Some students literally blossom with this individualized attention. Preceptors also benefit from the relationship with the student. Students are a stimulus and reinforce the SNP's feelings about their expertise and value.

MAKING THE EXPERIENCE SUCCESSFUL

We all talk about setting goals, but sometimes do not follow through. For our part, we had to be very clear about what we expected to accomplish with this experience. We began with the general goal that students would have a chance to actually participate in some areas of management, not simply observe or simulate them. Our second general goal was that students would appreciate the role of the registered nurse in a long-term care setting. Whether the students ever considered long-term care nursing as a personal choice, we hoped that they would carry with them into their various careers a positive view of this role in nursing.

After these general goals were determined, we wrote specific objectives for the clinical experience. One goal was to establish objectives related to each of the major unit topics covered in the management theory class that the students took in the quarter immediately preceding their management experience. Objectives included completion of a staff teaching project, evaluation of nursing assistants, delegation of tasks to nursing assistants, and collaboration with others on the health care team. Some of these objectives have become so well-established in the facility that staff are asking for specific educational topics and look forward to the presence of students in this role. From the beginning, we have revised our clinical objectives for this experience to reflect increased incorporation of a broad range of management concepts in practice.

CHOOSING SPECIFIC SETTING

Although we had already decided to use nursing homes for this experience, we did not know which homes. We are fortunate, however, that our geographic area has many nursing homes and formulated the following criteria to guide our choices:

1. Each facility had to have a registered nurse who could serve as a SNP during the time the student would be there. Because we believed in the unique role of the registered nurse in the nursing home, we believed it was essential that the student have a registered nurse as a preceptor.
2. Administrative staff, especially the director of nursing, needed to strongly support the program. We believed that if key people did not support what we were planning, the staff would not either.
3. We wanted to have more than one registered nurse in the facility available as a preceptor. We recognized that there would be sick days, vacation days, and just plain burnout. If there were more than one preceptor, we felt that the preceptors could "spell" each

other and provide mutual support. This was our ideal, but turned out to not always be possible. We still prefer it.

Although we had developed relationships with some nursing homes for our fundamentals students, we needed additional relationships. We called, visited, talked to nursing administrators and staff development coordinators, and explored the facilities. One facility with many positive attributes was in the midst of major organizational changes and we (facility staff and faculty) agreed that this was not the time to add students to the mix. However, we are keeping in contact and believe that this might someday be an excellent resource. Of the new sites developed since we started, one was opened to us via a preceptor from one facility taking a new position at another facility.

SELECTING STAFF NURSES FOR PRECEPTORS

How do we select the staff nurses who will serve as preceptors? We *don't!!* We provide the staff development coordinators or director of nursing with suggested criteria and ask them to select the nurses they believe to be suited to the role. Suggested criteria include: that the staff nurse like working with students, have good communication skills (be able to "talk students through" experiences and communicate how they make decisions), be a good role model (especially with regard to nurse-physician interactions), be honest with the student, be an expert in terms of organization and prioritization of resident care, be willing and able to share rationale for planning and intervention, demonstrate genuine caring for the residents' well-being, and possess experience and knowledge of the patient care area (Hsieh & Knowles, 1990; Lewis, 1986). In most cases the nurses chosen have been well-suited to the preceptor role.

PRECEPTOR PREPARATION

The literature clearly states that preceptors need preparation for the role (Limon, Bargagliotti, & Spencer, 1982). Shoreline preceptors initially received two eight-hour days, spaced one week apart. The first day was an overview of the management theory course, the second the "how to's" of being a preceptor. Because it was difficult to carve that much time out of the nurses' schedules and because it was expensive to provide two full days, the preparation is now provided in a one-day workshop. This includes a brief overview of management theory interwoven with applications of the theory in the nursing home setting and examples of how the preceptor can best assist the student in some typical situations. Topics included are an exploration of the roles of instructor, staff nurse preceptor, and nursing student; teaching/learning theory; principles of feedback and evaluation; and the opportunity to role-play some potential situations (Limon, Bargagliotti, & Spencer, 1982).

After the first year, an instructor involved in the preceptorship experience concluded that we needed to provide the preceptors with a handbook that would include all handouts provided during the preceptor preparation and give the preceptors a place to keep their ongoing records during a specific clinical period. The handbook has proven to be a useful and appreciated tool.

From the beginning, we knew that periodic "updates" would be required to allow preceptors to share problems and solutions, to provide new information, and to promote enthusiasm. To date, only one "official" update has been held.

We have attempted to provide some rewards and recognition to those nurses who serve as preceptors. The college provides them with a special name tag that adds "Shoreline Preceptor" to their title. Each facility that has preceptors is provided with a library card for the college library for use by the facility staff. Preceptors are also invited to attend our nursing continuing education events at reduced rates or no charge (depending on the event).

EVALUATING THE PRECEPTOR EXPERIENCE

Evaluation of the experience has been ongoing. We have elicited feedback from students, preceptors, facility nursing administration, and faculty. As we have become clearer in regard to our objectives and more effective in preparing the students for the experience, we have seen the students' response improve. They are now moving actively into the management role, expressing their understanding of how these concepts will transfer to other settings, and stating that they now appreciate the role of the registered nurse in the nursing home.

Preceptors provide feedback for individual student progress, as well as determining whether students have met individual objectives.

Faculty provide assistance and support to them in this role. Examples of both positive and negative evaluation statements have been developed to help the preceptors as they struggle with providing feedback. Preceptors have also been able to help us identify those areas that need strengthening for all students. Preceptors have stated that the new role is challenging and interesting and provides impetus for their own professional growth.

Faculty members have adapted to the new role of working through preceptors instead of directly with students, although it has been easier for some than for others. Changes have been made in the way students are oriented based on faculty identification of problems that students had. Additional written suggestions for activities to meet course objectives have lessened student anxiety. Faculty have also learned to accept preceptor turnover, preceptor burnout, and the ongoing need for preceptor training and update.

ANNOTATED BIBLIOGRAPHY

Chickarella, B.G., & Lutz, W.J. (1981). Professional nurturance: Preceptorships for undergraduate nursing students. *American Journal of Nursing, 81*(1), 107–109.
Preceptors were used in a final clinical rotation for students from Capital University to assist with role transition and counteracting the effects of "reality shock." Advantages included professional nurturance of the student by the preceptor, exposure to everyday practice and frustrations, and opportunity to work with solving problems of practice. Disadvantages included the time required of preceptors, difficulty with faculty evaluation of student performance, and unpredictable events such as the absence of a preceptor. Overall they recommend this experience.

Cotugna, N., & Vickery, C.E. (1990). Rewarding facility preceptors. *Nurse Educator 15*(4), 21–22.
Rewards to facility preceptors are largely intangible and include professional stimulation, contribution to the profession, professional pride, and bolstering enthusiasm. In addition, tangible rewards were designed. These included: a journal club organized by students, professional literature reviews done by students and shared with preceptors, lay literature reviews to assist preceptors in their teaching functions, clinical case study presentations by students, departmental seminars presented by the school for preceptors, access to book ordering, and library privileges and computer access.

Diers, D. (1990). Learning the art and craft of nursing. *American Journal of Nursing, 90*(1), 64–65.
This essay presents aspects of nursing as an art and supports the use of preceptors to socialize students into this significant arena of the nursing role. The author's delineation of the art of nursing provides stimulus to a wider view.

Dobbs, K.K. (1988). The senior preceptorship as a method for anticipatory socialization of baccalaureate nursing students. *Journal of Nursing Education, 27*(4), 167–171.
This research study supported the effectiveness of a senior preceptorship experience as a method for promoting anticipatory socialization to the working role of professional nurses. Changes occurred in role expectations and self-image. Corwin's Nursing Role Conception Scale was used.

Goldenburg, D. (1988). Preceptorship: A one-to-one relationship with a triple "P" rating. *Nursing Forum, 23*(1), 10–15.
A review of what is included in a preceptorship experience, benefits for all participants, and disadvantages of preceptorships. The author suggests that a reward mechanism for preceptors is essential and makes some suggestions of how this might be accomplished.

Hsieh, N.L., & Knowles, D.W. (1990). Instructor facilitation of the preceptorship relationship in nursing education. *Journal of Nursing Education, 29*(6), 262–268.
A research study that examined the development of the preceptor relationship. Three questions were addressed: what are the specific elements essential to the development of the preceptorship relationship? what is the role of the instructor in facilitating the developing preceptorship relationship?; and what are the variables affecting the developing preceptorship relationship? Seven commonly occurring themes were identified as important aspects of the developing relationship.

Lewis, K.E. (1986). What it takes to be a preceptor. *Canadian Nurse, 82*(12), 18–19.
A brief overview of suggestions for the preceptor. It includes ways that the preceptor may make this a more valuable experience for the student. Interpersonal relationships and communication are emphasized.

Limon, S., Bargagliotti, L.A., & Spencer, J.B. (1982). Providing preceptors for nursing students: What questions should you ask? *Journal of Nursing Administration, 12*(6), 16–17.
Suggestions for the nursing administrator to consider when asked to have staff participate as preceptors for nursing students. Emphasis is on establishing guidelines and direction before the experience begins.

Pierce, A.G. (1991). Preceptorial students' view of their clinical experience. *Journal of Nursing Education, 30*(6), 244–249.
Students responded to an anonymous questionnaire in regard to their clinical experience. Two themes emerged from the data: what students desire from their experience and the factors that influenced preceptorial experiences. There were differences found between first and last preceptorial clinical experiences.

Scheetz, L.J. (1989). Baccalaureate nursing student preceptorship programs and the development of clinical competence. *Journal of Nursing Education, 28*(1), 29–35.
One of the goals of clinical preceptorship may be to develop the student's level of competence beyond that of traditional baccalaureate nursing students. A summer preceptorship was developed. Results of the study indicated that students who

were participating in a preceptorship experience increased their problem solving, application of theory to practice, and psychomotor skill performance more than did students who worked as nursing assistants.

Yonge, O., & Profetto-McGrath, J. (1990). Coordinating a preceptorship program. *Canadian Nurse, 86*(9), 30–31.

The many difficulties in establishing and coordinating a preceptorship program are discussed. Negotiating placements, setting the terms of the preceptorship and coping with the problems that arise are all a part of the responsibility.

PART IV

Computers in the Classroom

14

Nursing Education and Computers: In Retrospect and Prospect

Patricia Tymchyshyn
Kathleen Lewis

COMPUTER BEGINNINGS

*I*t's been almost a quarter of a century since the first educational computer lessons were developed by Marianne Bitzer on the PLATO educational computer system. Parkland College's Nursing Department was the first Associate Degree nursing program to participate in research done on the use of computer assisted instruction (CAI) to teach nursing via PLATO. Today there are few Associate Degree nursing programs who do not or are not interested in using computers in nursing education.

In response to the National League for Nursing's call for texts relating personal experiences in the growth of Associate Degree nursing, this chapter is written from the author's experiences in the development and spread of computers in nursing education. It begins with CAI developed on mainframes, based in collegiate classrooms, and ends with students using CAI on laptop computers to teach patients in the community.

PLATO at Parkland

Tymchyshyn's computer roots began in 1968 with PLATO, a state-of-the-art mainframe instructional system, located at the University of Illinois in Urbana. Marianne Bitzer, a nursing instructor and wife of PLATO inventor Donald Bitzer, completed the development of 22 PLATO III lessons for a hospital-based maternity nursing course, and enlisted the assistance of Parkland College's nursing faculty in evaluating PLATO's applicability to a community college program. Bitzer's lessons presented materials in a manner that required students to seek, sort, organize, interpret, and apply information. The computer judged words and word phrases, provided feedback, and allowed learner-controlled branching through the lessons. Evaluation showed that instruction could be completed in one-third the time of traditional methods, but there was no difference in achievement compared to traditional instructional methods. Attitudes of students were positive and they enjoyed using the lessons and generally preferred it to lecture discussion methodology. Parkland's faculty was excited about the new technology and incorporated it into their maternal child health curriculum.

Developing New PLATO Lessons

By 1972, however, the lessons were no longer available as PLATO evolved into its next evolutionary stage, becoming PLATO IV. The hardware changes were extraordinary. Response time was .2 second, over 2,000 characters could be displayed on the screen, with 256 characters immediately available. The plasma display panel could simultaneously show computer-generated graphics with text and color slides. Other marvels included random accessed audio as well as touch panels for learner input. If Parkland wished to continue using PLATO, it was clear that new nursing lessons would have to be developed that incorporated PLATO's impressive instructional delivery capabilities.

Parkland's nursing director was a strong PLATO advocate and encouraged her faculty in lesson development. Tymchyshyn and another faculty member, Jean Helper, enjoyed using PLATO and applied for federal funding. They were awarded a $250,000 Health Education and Welfare grant to develop and evaluate PLATO IV lessons for nursing education. The grant included monies for a PLATO computer laboratory with 24 terminals connected to the mainframe at the University of Illinois. They designed lessons that used the computer's ability to (1) store, retrieve, analyze and interpret data; (2) support drill and practice, tutorials, simulations and gaming strategies; and (3) vary presentation of information through graphics, animation, color slides, and audio. It was a designer's delight. If PLATO couldn't do what lessons authors wanted today, its developers would create it tomorrow. A very popular lesson incorporated a gaming strategy to teach students about the changes that occurred in fetal circulation after birth. It used graphics and animation to illustrate the fetus's circulatory structure. Students, as captains of oxygen carrying vessels, used a touch screen to navigate through critical "ports" in the circulation process. They were judged on their ability to identify fetal circulatory structure and purpose. Help sequences consisted of color slides representative of true fetal anatomy. A total of fifteen lessons were developed.

Program evaluation illustrated that the computer lessons saved time, successfully replacing lecture, were useful in preparing students for clinical practice, and increased opportunities for independent study. Students once again preferred the computer to other instructional mediums, selecting simulations, inquiry, and gaming as their favorite lesson strategies. There was no difference in achievement when compared to lecture and discussion presentations. Students were PLATO's greatest proponents. They wanted more lessons without delay. Although maternal child health nursing faculty eventually accepted the computer as an integral part of the teaching environment, it was difficult for them to give up lectures and prepare discussion sessions based on PLATO lessons.

Concurrently, faculty in biology, chemistry, English, accounting, foreign language, and mathematics developed or used programs designed at other PLATO sites. They grew in sophistication and number. By the late 1970s, PLATO was institutionalized at Parkland. Over a third of the disciplines at the college used the computer lab for classes or independent study. Control Data Corporation contracted with the University of Illinois to market PLATO lessons nationwide.

SPREADING THE WORD

There was a newfound excitement in teaching. Technology had sparked Tymchyshyn's curiosity and she became committed not only to developing CAI programs, but to sharing her experiences with others. She joined other nurses, educators, and computer specialists in the presentation of information through computer workshops and conferences across the United States and internationally. PLATO nursing lessons and evaluations were presented at the first International Computers in Nursing Symposium held in London in 1983. Nurses and computer scientists from over 20 countries met to share their knowledge and goals, and to plan strategies for the future development and integration of computers in nursing. This information was organized into a publication entitled, *The Impact of Computers on Nursing, An International Review*, that described computer applications related to nursing records, patient monitoring, community-based care, drug management, nursing service and management, education, and research.

Nurses returned home to encourage our colleagues to increase their involvement with this new technology. The National League for Nursing (NLN) initiated a Forum and the American Nurse's Association, a Council on Computer Applications in Nursing. Tymchyshyn served on the NLN computer board and the ANA task force on education helping to organize conferences and workshops to (1) assist nurses in learning about all applications of computers in nursing, (2) provide a forum for sharing new development, and (3) establish guidelines for computer integration into the curriculum. The interest was enormous!

Tymchyshyn was then asked to design computer and other visual media under a W. K. Kellogg grant at California State University's Statewide Nursing Program. Parkland's nursing faculty continued to use the maternity lessons, but designed nothing new. Nursing students, however, were able to expand their use of computers in other college courses, such as communications, biology, foreign language, and chemistry. In 1984, Lewis became interested in PLATO's ability to assess student knowledge and developed test items for all the medical-surgical courses.

FROM MAINFRAMES TO MICROS

For many academic institutions, the cost of accessing educational lessons through mainframes was too high. Microcomputers were gaining in popularity and became an attractive and affordable alternative. Once more nursing was challenged to develop new lessons for a different type of hardware and software delivery system. Authoring systems designed for micros could not only support the same lesson strategies, but offer color for background and foreground applications. They also supported animation, sound, and screen prints. One major dilemma was whether to purchase and design programs for Apple or IBM since the lessons were not interchangeable across these two major types of micro hardware. Both Lewis and Tymchyshyn felt that IBM would support post secondary institutions and encouraged faculty at Parkland and Statewide, respectively, to purchase IBM hardware. Statewide began development of software for nursing support courses in areas such as pathophysiology. Authors with mainframe experience began developing software for micros as well as commercial vendors. The availability of nursing software grew rapidly.

Motivating with Micros

Although Parkland maintained its PLATO classroom for collegewide use, faculty began adding microcomputers to individual department labs throughout the college. Nursing acquired four IBM micros and purchased 12 software programs. However, it wasn't until the late 1980s that Parkland's nursing administration became committed to the use of microcomputer technology. With the director's support, Lewis became the microcomputer resource person and was able to motivate an increased number of faculty to evaluate software for their courses. It soon became clear that four computers were inadequate to meet the needs of 24 faculty and nearly four hundred students. The nursing department chair encouraged Lewis and Tymchyshyn, who had returned to Parkland, to seek funding through the Helene Fuld Trust Fund. The department was awarded $50,000 for development of a nursing computer laboratory consisting of 14 microcomputers and a beginning software library for each course. Most software was purchased for the purpose of instruction (e.g., simulations, tutorials, assessments, and remedial programs). Each course had two hours per student allotted, weekly.

Excitement about new uses of computers in nursing education was running high once more. However, new ideas need new funding sources. The college provided internal grants and supported the use of nursing budget funds for computer support. Lewis was named Administrative Fellow for Integration of Computer Technology in Nursing. Together, she and Tymchyshyn initiated a software project to learn the use of Quest, an authoring system from Allen Communications. Three lessons were developed in medical-surgical nursing.

Other faculty became interested in test authoring systems and began designing their own micro-based computer assessments. Soon an interactive video system was purchased for use in all courses. Some lessons were used as part of a classroom presentation, others for supplementing clinical experience and others as assigned coursework. Tymchyshyn began teaching a computers in nursing course for continuing education, introducing students to nursing applications of spreadsheets and database and word-processing packages. Computer use had snowballed.

NEW DIRECTIONS

Parkland nursing's newest venture is once again being supported by a Helene Fuld Trust Grant. Instead of students using computers in a lab at the college, the students will take laptop computers to teach clients in community settings. Faculty believe that the computer augments the students' ability to provide patient education. Although each nursing course has a clinical teaching component, students are by no means proficient teachers. Computer software offers consistent, well-developed content that can be used by students in presentation of information.

The first use of the laptops will be in a clinical experience with the elderly in their homes. In this course, students visit clients to assess their independent living skills and to provide health promotion information. Students and clients will use computer software to assess health knowledge about nutrition. Together, they will select nutritional modules that interest the client and meet their needs.

Another community setting is an obstetrician's office. Students will work with nursing staff to assist clients in using a computerized contraceptive risk assessment and birth control preference survey. Clients, following completion of a CAI module on their preferred contraceptive, will meet with the student and nurse to discuss their contraceptive needs and problems. Tymchyshyn has received state funding for this software development project.

CONCLUSION

Looking back over the past 25 years' experiences, it is clear how fortunate Parkland's nursing faculty was to be involved in the formative years of CAI on both mainframe and micro. This innovation sparked curiosity and generated excitement in both teaching and instructional development. However, if an innovation is to be successful, it must have administrative support and advocacy of individuals who are willing to spend time nurturing its growth. When Parkland had support of nursing administration and faculty advocacy, its computer use flourished. Today, faculty and administration are both involved in and committed to the exciting new prospects of computers in nursing education.

15

Innovation in the Classroom: How to Meet the Technological Challenge

Ellen R. Bramoweth

*T*here are many disciplines that take great pride in stating, "the technological advances which have occurred in our area over the past ten years have been remarkable." In the health care field, however, we cannot make such a claim. For if we did, we would be speaking of things outdated, often no longer in use.

The knowledge-based technology associated with medicine, nursing, and health care change at such a rapid pace that we speak of significant advances with technological applications occurring on a continuous basis. This ever-changing situation creates somewhat of a dichotomy for those in nursing education. On the one hand, it provides a stimulating clinical arena that allows student nurses "hands-on" experience with all the specialized procedures and equipment. On the other hand, it creates a sharp contrast to the manner in which didactic, theoretical, content-focused instruction is presented in the classroom.

The main reason for this contrast is that while many faculty have been able to keep up with the clinical advances, they have not changed, in any fashion, the manner in which classroom instruction is conducted. Most instructors stand in front of the classes and speak to the students, using some assistance from an overhead projector or slide projector. The instructor will typically have notes to use, often handwritten, or now perhaps neatly typed on the word processor. If a student needs clarification on a point made several "pages" ago, the instructor will shuffle through the papers until the content is located. This process strands the faculty in the dark ages of teaching techniques.

Imagine for a moment walking into a classroom with no notes in your hand, no stack of papers used for the presentation or lecture. At the front of your room you have access to a computer, video cassette recorder/player, video disk player, a video pad camera capable of projecting all types of images from a transparency, to a page out of a text or current journal, to a single slide. The room is equipped with a large screen to display the material determined to best enhance the content of your lecture.

To many faculty, this image strikes terror into their hearts. They have only begun to master the intricacies of their word processors and are frequently frustrated trying to get the overhead projector to work in a consistent manner. As the faculty adopt new text books, they spend hours revising lecture content to maintain consistency. The thought of being thrust into the world of high-tech teaching is not viewed with enthusiastic anticipation.

Return to the imagined classroom. To make the scene more attractive, imagine that you have been trained to use all of the equipment made available to you. You have been assisted by experts in the field of computer and audio-video application. You began by developing one lecture series using software and techniques which added elements to your presentation never before thought possible.

But most importantly, after your first series of presentations, you have seen the response of the students. Not only were they alert, stimulated, and challenged in the classroom, but they came to you with reports of how they were able to apply this information in a more meaningful manner while working directly with patients in clinical settings.

It is for this last reason that nurse educators must be willing to meet the technological challenge in the classroom. We have a responsibility to provide the most current theoretical concepts in the most current, effective manner.

Many questions arise as to the needed hardware and software to implement such a program. Colleges across the nation have equipment currently on hand that would allow application of many of these techniques in the classroom. Other departments have monies available for equipment purchase, but have never considered changing from standard appliances such as overhead projectors to newer, more advanced items. Faculty must take the initiative to seek out current resources available to them.

The most important aspect involved in being able to implement a technologically sophisticated program is having the support personnel available to assist in the training of faculty in the creative use of the equipment. Without this support structure, faculty will meet unnecessary frustrations, which will quickly undermine the most committed intentions. Therefore, word must be spread to our college administrators not to let their investment in hardware and software be wasted. The most effective utilization would include further investment in highly qualified personnel.

I have been most fortunate at Mesa Community College, which is part of the Maricopa Community College District, in Arizona, to have available to me the very best personnel and equipment. This has helped make my transition to using technology in my classroom teaching rewarding and relatively painless.

I was able to demonstrate much of the equipment and the application of techniques during my presentation at the National League for Nursing's Council of Associate Degree Programs Annual Meeting and 40th Anniversary Celebration. This demonstration highlighted computer-aided presentations and use of the video pad camera.

With computer-aided presentations, the instructor's notes are placed in the computer for better organization and quick access. Lecture notes appear on the computer screen visible to the instructor. Methods of outlining and organizing content that would not be possible with printed pages make access to information more simple.

Each computer screen has "buttons" or controls that send commands to equipment used during the lecture, such as the video disk player (laserdisc). By moving the cursor (mouse) to the button on the screen, the instructor is able to start and stop the video player, without interrupting the flow of the lecture. It is possible to access multiple images simply through clicks on the buttons.

Additionally, text may be superimposed over the video images. Instead of using a pointer or light beam to point out significant sections of the image, the computer can be used to delineate the specific area. Definitions, outlines, or sections of text can also be generated through the computer and displayed on the large screen for student viewing. This can be prepared prior to lecture, or this feature can be used spontaneously during a presentation, to help clarify a point, reinforce proper spelling of terms, or pose questions.

The computer can be used for sounds as well as images. It is possible to access sounds that may be part of a laserdisc program. It is also possible to capture and present sounds through use of the computer program itself, without use of video disk or audio tape players. In this manner, pronunciation of medical terms, as well as sounds useful in teaching assessment skills (i.e., heart and breath sounds) can be generated in your classroom presentation.

Application of the computer-aided instruction is made more simple by the use of icons located on the screen viewed by the instructor. These visual cues help make the switch from one technique to another.

The video pad camera was also demonstrated during the NLN presentation. The pad camera allows any printed material such as photographs, slides, books, typed or handwritten pages, and small objects to be viewed on a TV monitor or large screen via projection. The large screen allows viewing of small details. This piece of equipment has been the most useful in changing classroom presentations. It allows for demonstration of equipment and techniques in a large classroom setting, so each student can see, in detail, what is being demonstrated.

The clarity and magnification of detail allow comparison of 1cc syringes (detecting the differences between 50 unit and 100 unit insulin syringes, for example). Placement of a triple lumen central venous catheter under the pad camera allows detailed inspection of the equipment by all students simultaneously, rather than the need to pass it around the room for the students' viewing.

The versatile nature of the pad camera allows use of existing transparencies, permitting use of previously developed teaching aids or aids provided by many textbook publishing companies. X-rays, models, and equipment can all be used with the pad camera.

The presentation utilized the computer-aided lecture, laserdisc (video disk) technology, and the video pad camera to demonstrate the use of technology in the classroom. Use of these techniques has brought challenge and stimulation to the faculty in its development, as well as rewards in its implementation, as measured by student response and feedback. Time was involved in making the switch to the new format. It was an investment well worth making.

16

Interactive Videodisc Technology in Nursing Education

Pam Springer
Carol Fountain

Several years ago, Boise State University, Boise, Idaho, made an institutional decision to implement computer technology throughout the university to the greatest extent possible. The university adopted an outcome statement on computer literacy for students, and each department within the university developed a philosophy on computer literacy for faculty and students. In general, the literacy statement said that a graduate of the university must be able to make use of the computer for tasks appropriate to his or her discipline.

The nursing department computer literacy statement, developed from the university literacy statement, was also based on several beliefs within the following framework: the computer should make jobs and work easier, not more difficult. The faculty thought computer technology should support various teaching methodologies. It was hoped that the faculty and students would be in control of the computer, not vice versa. Specifically, it was the faculty's goal that the computers would support teachers and students in efforts to provide and receive education.

The interest in computers of the nursing department faculty varied widely. Some faculty expressed no interest (would not even turn the computer on, and in fact, used the computer as a bulletin board) and had to be dragged "kicking and screaming" to a computer. On the other hand, there was a small group of very computer-literate members who already had programming skills. That small group of computer-literate faculty formed the nucleus of the department of nursing computer committee. The computer committee decided that, to implement the computer literacy statement of the university, all faculty in the department should become computer-literate. One goal of the computer committee, therefore, was to assist in increasing interest and skills of those who had less or no computer literacy. Computer games during faculty lunch hour were instituted. Gaining interest in the games soon spread to an interest in computers and additional software for computers. As the nursing department faculty became more computer-literate, the computer committee began to develop an interest in additional technology available using computers, including exploring the increased use of technology in the nursing curricula. Although the committee had heard about the possibilities of interactive video technology, committee members did not have much knowledge of or experience with it.

In response, the nursing department chair attended a national technology conference, viewed an interactive video demonstration, and related her experience with the technology there to the computer committee. The interactive video company was contacted by the nursing department for a demonstration. The computer committee arranged the presentation on use of interactive video and had the entire faculty view the presentation. The presentation involved treating a patient in an automobile accident. Faculty at the presentation were easily involved in the interactive program, and became very interested in the technology.

Unfortunately, this interest waned as the teaching responsibilities and meeting schedules filled up faculty time. Computer committee members, however, were still interested and continued to pursue applications of the newer technology. Finally, their interest in acquiring and using this newer technology met with success.

DEFINITIONS

Interactive videodisc programs use the interaction of a computer (almost any computer) combined with the clarity and accessibility of videodisc pictures. The user interacts with the computers and obtains a response depending on answers given, similar to computer-assisted instruction (CAI). Combined with this interaction are the pictures, either still or motion, from the videodisc. The interaction comes when the individual makes selections from the screen, usually by touching the screen, and progresses through the program at his or her own pace and desired pattern. Even computer-phobic people can accept new videodisc technology fairly easily because it involves a video player. Most people have at home a video tape player connected to a TV.

FUNDING

Nursing department funding was needed to implement the use of interactive video technology. The department of nursing, thus, wrote a grant proposal to the Helen Fuld Foundation, and was funded for approximately $46,000. The Fuld Foundation is a philanthropic foundation that gives grants to nursing schools and other allied health schools. The department was then able to purchase the equipment to implement interactive videodisc programs into the curriculum. Other schools interested in acquiring similar technology should consider grant sources such as the Fuld Foundation. In addition, other schools should investigate local businesses including computer technology companies, and have the school fund-raising group offer advice on raising funds. The grant funds allowed the establishment of six student stations and one faculty work station. The student stations are for student use, to view the interactive programs. Students can view programs individually or in small groups. The faculty work station, with an authoring system loaded on, is the station used by faculty to develop programs, or to make alterations in current programs or discs.

EQUIPMENT

The following is a list of equipment:

Student station:
- *Computer.* IBM compatible computer (286 or higher is recommended)—16 meghz CPU, 640K ram 40 meg hard drive (minimum

of 40 meg memory recommended due to demands of several programs), 1.4 floppy drive, 3.5-inch disk drive. Because of the recent developments in the technology, 386 computers are now almost one half of the price they were one year ago, and would be an excellent choice for student stations.

- *Laser disc player.* The Pioneer laser disc player is compatible with the computer and Visage system. Other common brands of laser disc players include Sony.
- *Touch-screen monitor.* The Visage system is a touch-screen system and requires a special monitor. Such a system is required in order to utilize a touch-screen interactive program. There are other touch-screen systems available, but Visage was found to be the best quality for the price.

Faculty work station:

- *Computer.* IBM compatible computer, 386 or higher CPU, 120 meg memory. The larger memory is because of the demands of the authoring system, other development software, and faculty developed programs that are in process and stored on the computer.
- *Laser disc player.* Laser disc player with hand control (see above).
- *Touch-screen monitor.* Touch-screen monitor (see above). A VGA or EGA graphics card is necessary to run most of the programs.

COST

The cost for the student and faculty work stations varies, with equipment as the initial and greatest cost. The newest model of computer available that fits the budget should be selected. Schools that have some current equipment should consider upgrading that equipment to keep costs lower. Be sure that the bid for purchase includes local support and service for the hardware purchased.

Technical assistance will probably be needed to set up a system. Instructional media centers frequently have technical and support personnel and those people can be of great assistance in developing a system. Technical support from companies is also a factor to consider; companies are usually very ready to answer questions if problems develop.

The interactive programs themselves range in price from $300 to $1,600 or more per program. The more expensive programs have, of course, more information and more options available in the course-ware. The $300 programs tend to be a videodisc only, with no computer interaction possible.

AUTHORING SYSTEM

The department of nursing computer committee decided that they also needed an authoring system. An authoring system is a computer program (software) that can incorporate multimedia in developing professional quality computer-based training or education programs. The multimedia programs engage the senses of sight, hearing, and touch in an educational program. The authoring system has the added capabilities of tracking and recording a learner's progress through the interactive program. The authoring system can be used to adapt the noninteractive discs. The system can also be used to adapt the commercial interactive videodiscs for another purpose. This adaptation is called repurposing. Repurposing a program allows more effective use of a disc, and it can be adapted to individual courses or curricula. Repurposing also can be used to keep information current. This is done by changing the text presented to the student, but continuing to use the pictures from the disc.

Our authoring system chosen was *Quest,* developed by Allen Communications of Salt Lake City, Utah. *Quest* was chosen as an authoring system over *ICON, TENCORE,* or several others because of the ease of use, graphics capability, and other advantages identified in the program. One brief warning, however—the *Quest* program is not a computer game that is mastered in 15 minutes. It takes work and effort to learn to utilize it quickly, but is fairly user-friendly.

The authoring system can also be used to develop CAI programs that are interactive, utilizing the touch-screen monitor. The programs can be developed by digitizing pictures, and including text, animation, and graphics. Digitized pictures are obtained by taking a picture of an object with a video camera, and, with special computer equipment and programs, transferring the picture to a computer graphic that can be incorporated into the CAI program. This requires special equipment that nursing programs do not need to purchase if media departments have such equipment. Again, the institutional media specialists should be involved in helping the faculty develop digitized pictures.

CRITERIA FOR PURCHASE

Several criteria were used to select interactive video discs (IVD) for purchase.

Subject Matter

Does the available subject matter suit the curriculum? If it is not an exact fit, can the program be repurposed? If the computer software can be rewritten to allow use of the video pictures, it may be a good investment. Frequently, an interactive video disc (IVD) can be repurposed so it can be used for several different courses.

Technical Support

Can the program be easily loaded and started? Does the company offer free technical support if problems arise?

Control

Controlling the program is an essential feature to consider when evaluating IVD. Is there progression to the program? Can students easily find their way around in the program? The program should be laid out logically and students should be able to move around it easily without having to complete long sessions. Students should be able to access the main menu and exit the screen at any point. Can students redo or review sections and control the amount of time spent on any screen? Unlike videotape, students can repeat material as many times as is necessary to master the content or may skip material if they are competent. The ability to repeat content on the screen brings the advantages of CAI combined with the clarity of video pictures.

Features

Important features are main menus, smooth screen transitions, touch areas, and making choices. The main menu should be comprehensive and list all of the selections available, including the ability to exit.

Because video disc pictures can be jerky or jittery when the motion stops, screen transitions should be smooth. The touch areas on the screen should be easily identifiable and large enough to touch. If the touch areas are small or hard to distinguish, students will become frustrated trying to get the computer to register the correct answer. Once choices are made, the selected choice should be distinguished by a changing color.

The nursing department at Boise State University (BSU) advocates IVD usage because it is a safe environment in which to practice. Intellectual skills and judgment can be practiced in an environment away from patients. Students can make decisions, try them out, and see the consequences, all in the safe environment of a computer or practice lab.

CURRENT USAGE

Therapeutic Communication, put out by the Fuld Institute for Technology in Nursing Education (FITNE), was the first IVD program purchased. This IVD program teaches therapeutic communication by teaching theory and utilizes vignettes to demonstrate communication techniques. At BSU, therapeutic communication is usually taught by demonstration and role playing. Even with this, when the *Therapeutic Communication* IVD is used, students generally have a positive experience. This IVD is used in clinical groups and also assigned out individually for students struggling with these concepts. Students can interact with patients as if they were the nurse. Students choose a response to what the patient on the IVD says. Based on the student's choice, the patient reacts and feedback is provided, all in a safe environment.

Nursing Decisions, also put out by FITNE, is another IVD used. This IVD follows a patient through having a cholecystectomy. Although this type of cholecystectomy surgery may be outdated, the determining concepts are not. The IVD begins with the admission assessment and continues through postoperative assessments. This IVD shows the thinking and decision-making process of the nurse. It allows students to "get inside the head of the nurse" to see how "real" nurses think and how they make decisions.

Another IVD used in the curriculum is *Ethical Dilemmas and Legal Issues in the Care of the Elderly,* from the American Journal of Nursing Company. This IVD utilizes four cases to cover legal/ethical issues such as advance directives, use of restraints, and code blue without a clear "do not resuscitate" order. To make these legal/ethical decisions, the students can utilize a library of terms, and consult an ethicist and an attorney. Students must clarify their values continually as they progress through the IVD, which also shows a variety of professionals with differing opinions, all of which are "right." Such complexity helps students struggle with their values, which tend to be "black and white," and forces them to reanalyze them. This program is used with clinical groups and also assigned individually.

To supplement limited maternal-child experiences we use Health Science Consortium's IVD *Managing the Experience of Labor and Delivery*. This realistic IVD allows students to participate in the entire labor and delivery experience. Students who use this IVD before they go into the delivery suite find that it heightens their focus on the role of the nurse once they are placed in the delivery experience with an actual patient.

Another IVD we use in our curriculum is *Disorders of the Nervous System: Motor*, from the University of Washington. This is an archival disc that had no computer software with it. Using *Quest*, a computer program was developed to control the videodisc. This made it possible to show unique clinical video pictures such as dolls eyes, absent corneal reflexes, and decerebrate posturing. The student can view assigned content as many times as needed to master the concepts.

CONCLUSION

Faculty interest has grown over the two-year period of IVD use. The core group helps to maintain this interest. The core group previews most IVDs and recommends purchase of IVDs for content areas not currently covered.

Drawbacks to implementing an IVD system are faculty time, equipment cost, and need for technical support. Benefits include being able to supplement limited clinical areas and experiences, being able to practice decision making in a safe environment, and versatility of IVDs. To put together a system requires a dedicated faculty, funding for hardware and software, and, most importantly, a never ending sense of humor.